Signs
and
Graphics
for
Health Care
Facilities

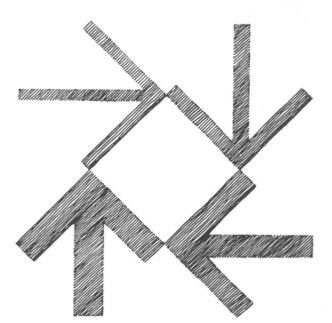

American Hospital Association
840 North Lake Shore Drive
Chicago, Illinois 60611

Library of Congress Cataloging in Publication Data

American Hospital Association.
  Signs and graphics for health care facilities.

    "AHA catalog no. 1262."
    Bibliography: p.
    Includes index.
    1. Hospitals—Design and construction. 2. Signs
and sign-boards. 3. Graphic arts—Technique.
I. Title. [DNLM: 1. Facilities design and construction. 2. Hospital administration. 3. Health
facilities. WX150 A511sd]
RA967.A47   1977a]   658.4'51   77-26180
ISBN 0-87258-179-9

AHA catalog no. 1262

© 1979 by the American Hospital Association
840 North Lake Shore Drive
Chicago, Illinois 60611

Printed in the U.S.A.
7M-12/78-6012

Printed by
Visual Images Inc.
Chicago, Illinois

CONTENTS

Foreword   v

CHAPTER **1**   **The Why and How of a Signs and Graphics System**   1

CHAPTER **2**   **Site Planning**   5
Planning and Identifying Approaches   7
Situating Parking Areas   12
Checklist for Site Planning   14

CHAPTER **3**   **Interior Planning**   17
Checklist for Interior Planning   20

CHAPTER **4**   **Data Collection**   23
Determining Uses and Conditions   25
Plotting the Information   26
Determining the Signs You Need   32
Checklist for Data Collection   34

CHAPTER **5**   **Choosing Messages and Media**   35
Terminology   35
Symbols and Pictographs   37
Color   40

CHAPTER **6**   **Choosing Signs**   41
Typeface   43
Letter Size   44
Layout   46
Placement   50

CHAPTER **7**   **Acquiring Signs**   51
Cost and Budgeting   52
Taking Bids and Ordering   53
Delivery   54
In-house Systems   54

CHAPTER **8**   **Numbering Systems**   55

CHAPTER **9**   **Maintaining the System**   61
Temporary Signs   61
Maintenance Procedures   62

Bibliography   63

Index   67

FOREWORD

Recognizing that health care facilities should have a readily understandable, coherent system of signs and graphics, the Society for Technical Communication, through the efforts of Jerilynn G. Sweeney, established a committee to work with the American Hospital Association to determine how best to encourage well-planned visual information systems in health care facilities. The committee concluded that the most useful product of its efforts would be a book that would explain the need for such a system and describe how to achieve a satisfactory one. Subsequently, an American Hospital Association Advisory Panel on Signposting for Hospitals was established to produce the book.

The American Hospital Association acknowledges with gratitude the efforts of the advisory panel. All of the members of the panel gave freely of their time and their knowledge to help plan and write the book. The members of the panel were:

Paul Arthur
Chairman of the Board
Newton Frank Arthur Christopher
Toronto, Ont., Canada

Susanne F. Batko
Assistant Director
Center for Urban Hospitals
American Hospital Association
Chicago, IL

Ernest W. Libman
Executive Director
San Luis Valley Health
  Maintenance Organization, Inc.
Alamosa, CO

Marilyn Ludwig
Public Relations
San Francisco, CA

Rex N. Olsen
Executive Editor and Associate Publisher
American Hospital Association
Chicago, IL

Gerald F. Oudens, AIA
Partner
Oudens + Knoop Architects
Washington, DC

Dorothy Saxner
Manager, Books and Newsletters
American Hospital Association
Chicago, IL

Jerilynn G. Sweeney
President
Identitia Inc.
Newburyport, MA

Marjorie E. Weissman
Senior Editor
American Hospital Association
Chicago, IL

In addition, special thanks are due to Jerilynn G. Sweeney, who prepared much of the technical information that appears here; to Gerald F. Oudens, who wrote the chapters on interior and exterior planning; to Marilyn Ludwig, who was the principal author; to Shevra Martin of Friesen International, Washington, DC, who did much of the early literature research; to Dorothy Saxner, who was instrumental in encouraging the Society for Technical Communication and the American Hospital Association to undertake the work; to Susanne F. Batko, who coordinated the project; to Marjorie E. Weissman, who edited the manuscript and prepared the book for publication; and to Walter Enck, graphic designer, Chicago, who made the illustrations.

1

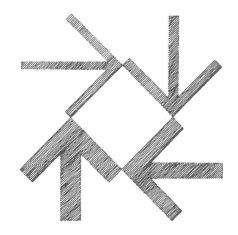

THE WHY AND HOW OF A SIGNS AND GRAPHICS SYSTEM

A coherent, logical, and easily understood system of informational signs and graphics in a hospital or other health care institution can make a substantial contribution to the smooth functioning of the institution and the satisfaction of its users. Among the many daily demands on hospital administrators, their time and effort are well spent in developing such a system. Therefore, this book was written to answer two questions: Why does a health care facility need such a system? How can the hospital administration go about developing it?

This introductory chapter is primarily an answer to the first question, Why? The remainder of the book provides answers to the second question, How? Although the book frequently refers to hospitals and the content has been directed primarily to them, the principles and many of the techniques discussed apply equally to other types of health care facilities, such as freestanding clinics and long-term care facilities.

Most of the book is about signs; nonetheless, signs are only one way of communicating information. Other ways include symbols, pictures, color, lighting, people, landscaping, and the architecture of the building itself. Information is also communicated by such items as the institution's logotype; its letterhead, billhead, and business cards; and external and internal newsletters—in short, all those things that make up the hospital's corporate identity.

Why a signs and graphics system at all? Because a thoughtfully planned system of informational signs and graphics can help people move to and through the hospital with a minimum of delay and anxiety. It can help get them where they need to be and tactfully steer them away from areas where they should not be. A good system also can reduce interruptions for the staff and thus help the hospital to function more efficiently.

Signs and graphics that give clear, consistent, tactful messages can do more than put people on the right path and keep them there; they can help get across the message that the institution and its personnel are concerned with the needs and anxieties of patients and visitors—that they want to help. On the other hand, a welter of confusing signs, incomprehensible terminology, and cardboard notices taped on walls can convey negative messages: "We think you're troublesome." "We have our own problems." "Don't bother us—we're just as confused as you are!"

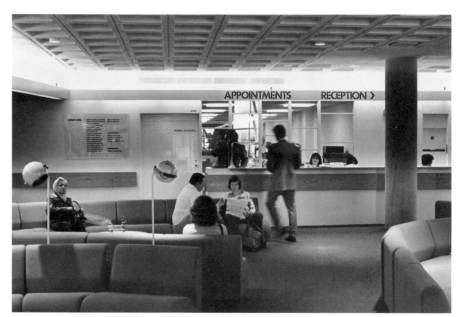

Photo: Courtesy Coco Raynes/Graphics, Inc. Architect: Payette Assoc., Inc.

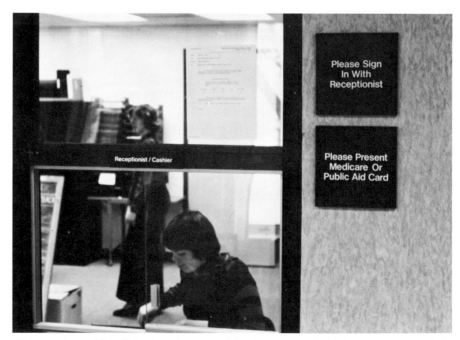

Signs and graphics that give clear, consistent messages help to assure users that the hospital wants to help them.

When and where do hospital users need information and directions? At every decision point in an individual's progress to and through the facility. These decision points are fewer if the user is escorted, and more if he is on his own. The system of informational signs and graphics should therefore perform at least four basic functions. It should (1) direct, (2) identify, (3) orient, and (4) provide additional information where needed.

These four basic functions serve different publics: the institution's patients; various types of visitors, such as patients' relatives and friends, delivery and service personnel, the police, and the press; and the medical, nursing, and other staff members and the volunteers. In addition, the hospital has an obligation to an even larger public — the community at large.

Of these publics, patients and their families and friends may need reassurance as much as they need information. They are in an unfamiliar environment, surrounded by strange faces, sights, and sounds. They may be frightened, disoriented, handicapped, apprehensive, or otherwise functioning at below-normal level. Information that is comprehensible and humanely given can help reassure them by restoring a sense of orientation and therefore control over their whereabouts.

Adapted from a chart by
E. Christopher Klumb Associates, New York City.
Hospital users need information and direction at every point in their progress to and through the facility. These decision points are fewer if users are escorted, more if they are alone.

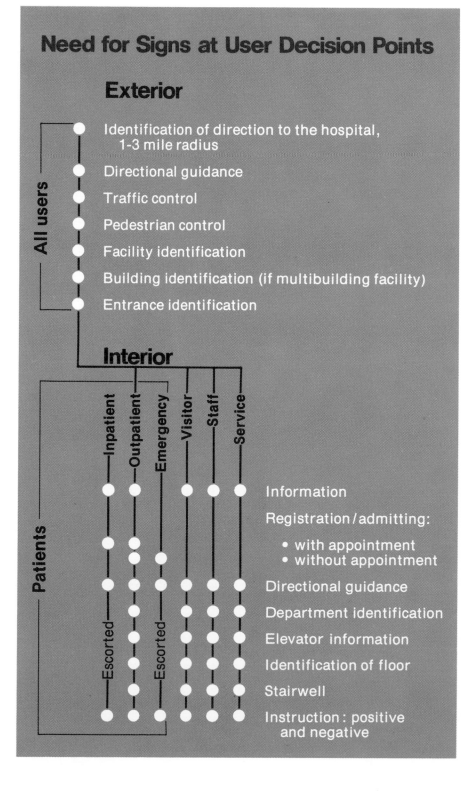

Need for Signs at User Decision Points

Exterior

All users
- Identification of direction to the hospital, 1-3 mile radius
- Directional guidance
- Traffic control
- Pedestrian control
- Facility identification
- Building identification (if multibuilding facility)
- Entrance identification

Interior

	Patients			Visitor	Staff	Service	
	Inpatient	Outpatient	Emergency				
Information	●	●		●	●	●	
Registration/admitting: • with appointment • without appointment	●	●	●				
Directional guidance	●	●	●	●	●	●	
Department identification		●	●	●	●	●	
Elevator information	●	●	●	●	●	●	
Identification of floor		●		●	●	●	
Stairwell		●	●	●	●	●	
Instruction: positive and negative	●	●	●	●	●	●	

(Inpatient: Escorted; Emergency: Escorted)

Staff members, too, need orientation and direction, at least at first. So do volunteers. Both groups have reason to value an effective information system as a time-saver, for persons who have trouble finding their way in the hospital will inevitably ask the help of the nearest person wearing a uniform or an identification badge.

Serving the community requires visibility in a literal sense; the hospital is obligated to let the community know where it is and how it is accessible. To someone bringing an accident victim to the hospital, for example, finding the right freeway exit and the emergency department entrance quickly is a matter of urgent necessity. A good signs and graphics system can help ensure that the hospital is clearly identified from all approaches and that people and vehicles get to the right entrances without confusion and delay.

How can the hospital administration go about developing a rational, coherent, functional system? This book is intended to demystify the process by providing detailed, step-by-step explanations of the decisions that must be made and the actions that must be taken. Also, the book includes tools that will help: checklists, illustrations, and technical information.

The process need not be complex or expensive, but it does require that the administration initially make the decision to commit time, effort, and money. Often it is possible to develop a system that incorporates some of the hospital's existing signs. Implementation of a system can be phased in over a brief or extended period, depending on the complexity of the system and the nature of the

problems. Because there inevitably will be signs, a flexible, well-thought-out system that allows for changes and additions is more economical than an ad hoc approach to sign acquisition.

The process outlined in this book is applicable to an existing facility as well as to one that is still on the drawing board. It can be used by a hospital administration that is committed to an existing physical plant and is without plans for any major alteration or expansion in the foreseeable future; by one planning minor or major alterations and/or additions; or by one anticipating the design and construction of an all-new facility.

A good system can help make the best of whatever exists. For example, in a plant that has been expanded by a process of random accretion over the years, it can help organize the flow of traffic to and through the various hospital wings or buildings.

If major alterations or additions are planned, the time is ideal for rethinking the signs and graphics system. A reappraisal at this time can suggest ways to avoid the

perpetuation of former mistakes and the means of linking the old facility with the new in such a way as to minimize possible confusion.

When a health care facility has a master plan, a master signs and graphics system is a worthwhile investment. In the case of an all-new facility, planning the system along with the new construction can help avoid some built-in ambiguities. If a major construction program is phased in over several years, the signs and graphics system can be phased in on a coordinated schedule and in the same way. The overall plans for the system are made, and the implementation is scheduled as construction or renovation is completed.

The study that is required to develop the system can itself suggest ways of solving problems. Outdoors, new walkways or shrubbery can guide people in the direction they should go. Inside, large planters can be effective as nonverbal signals. A professional such as an architect, who is accustomed to taking a comprehensive view of facility needs, can sometimes suggest relatively simple ways of rerouting traffic into desired patterns by making minor physical modifications.

Ideally, the building and its site should be effective communicators. A building that, through its design, steers traffic in the desired directions and away from undesirable ones requires fewer signs, maps, and verbal directions.

2

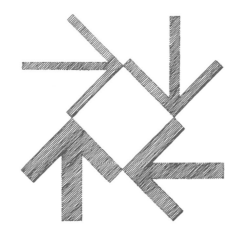

SITE PLANNING

When starting a new building program, a major building addition, or remodeling, hospital administrators and their architects and interior designers have a unique opportunity to include in the design a logical system of informational signs and graphics. Communication of desirable traffic patterns, that is, the way in which the facility is meant to be used and, therefore, the way in which it is designed, starts with site planning and building design.

Basic planning should take into account such considerations as location of building entrances relative to site access, onsite drives, and parking areas, as well as topography, orientation, views, organization of building elements, and architectural massing. The main entrance drive should be physically and visually separated from parking areas. Shrubbery, lighting, and other design elements, used singly or together, will accomplish this separation.

Planning should make desired movement patterns inevitable, because inevitability is the most effective way of ensuring intended use. For example, if visitors ought to enter the building through the main entrance, then visitor parking should be located on the main entrance side of the building; if the emergency department entrance is beyond the main entrance, there will be conflicts between emergency and visitor traffic.

A person making his initial visit to the hospital looks for directions and is alert to both explicit and implicit signs. In a suburban or rural setting or other open site, the hospital building complex itself can be the first "sign," if it is visible from the road. The often-

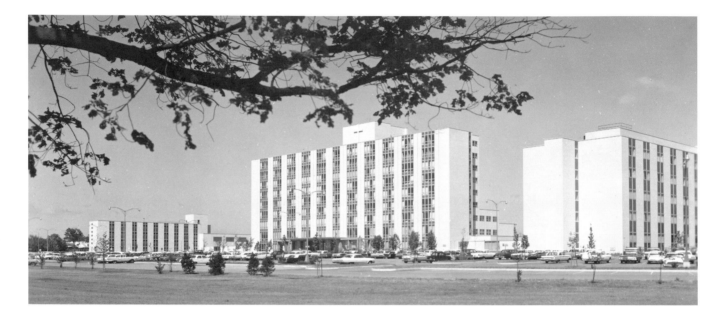

characteristic massing of a hospital's facilities can also help tell the visitor that he has arrived. Zoning and site restrictions on an urban site are major influences on massing and design, but even with these limitations, the building design usually can be helpful in identifying the hospital for what it is.

Signs and other means of communication are required to the extent that basic planning has not conveyed the necessary information.

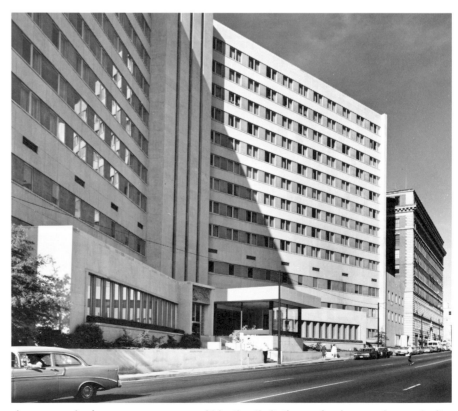

In open suburban areas or even within the limitations of urban zoning and site restrictions, the characteristic design of a hospital can usually be helpful in identifying it.

Planning and Identifying Approaches

In planning for site approach and traffic control, it is necessary to consider the main hospital entrance, visitor parking, medical staff parking, employee parking, the service yard, and the emergency department entrance area, as well as the location of and the access to other facilities on the site, such as a medical office building, a nurses' residence, or minimal-care domiciliary facilities. If a separate outpatient department entrance is considered necessary, it and related parking must also be taken into account.

If the main entrance is designed to *look* like a main entrance and if it can be seen from the vehicular or pedestrian approach route, the visitor will identify the entrance drive as the one that leads to the main entrance.

Similarly, a service yard with a loading dock, liquid oxygen storage, mechanical equipment plant, or other recognizable features will identify the area for service vehicles and discourage other visitors.

The identity of the hospital can be reinforced by a sign at the first site-entrance drive. If the hospital is set far back on its site and cannot easily be seen from the road, the first identifying sign should be located *before* the entrance drive and the second sign *at* the drive.

Main Entrance Drive

The main entrance drive logically should be the first drive off the approach road. However, site development does not always permit this. Often a hospital is planned and situated so that the service and emergency department en-

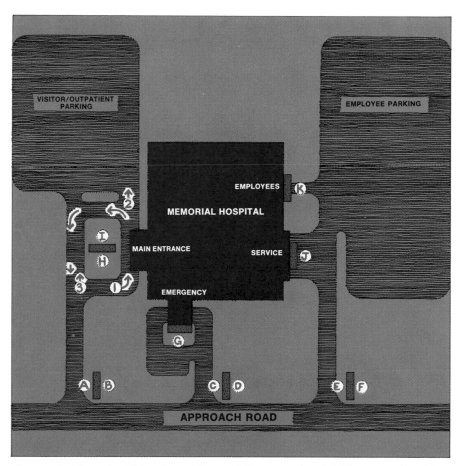

Approach drives should be planned to avoid the necessity of driving around parking areas.

A. Memorial Hospital
←Main Entrance
←Visitor Parking
↑Emergency
↑Service Entrance

B. Memorial Hospital
→Main Entrance
→Visitor Parking

C. Memorial Hospital
←Emergency
↑Service Entrance

D. Memorial Hospital
→Emergency
↑Main Entrance
↑Visitor Parking

E. Memorial Hospital
←Service Entrance

F. Memorial Hospital
→Service Entrance
↑Emergency
↑Main Entrance
↑Visitor Parking

G. Emergency

H. Memorial Hospital
→Main Entrance
↑Visitor Parking

I. Memorial Hospital
←Main Entrance
↑Exit

J. Service Entrance

K. Employee Entrance

1. Vehicular traffic should move in a counterclockwise direction past the main entrance.

2. Visitor parking should be beyond the drop-off point.

3. Traffic moving directly to the parking area should not interfere with the drop-off point.

trance drives precede the main entrance drive. This arrangement keeps all drives as short as possible and avoids the need for them to skirt the visitor parking area, which should be located beyond the main entrance. If the first drive encountered is the service entrance drive, additional signs should be posted to indicate that the emergency department and main entrance drives lie beyond. Similarly, if the next entrance is to the emergency department, for example, a second sign should indicate that the main entrance drive is further on. Signs should be placed at all decision points along the various entrance routes.

If the limitations of the site are such as to make it impossible to accommodate visitors' cars, a situation that often prevails in an urban setting, signs at entrance drives should indicate where visitors can park, rather than only prohibit parking by means of such legends as "Doctors Parking Only" or "Service Vehicles Only."

If the first drive encountered is the service entrance drive, additional signs should be posted to indicate that the emergency department and main entrance drives lie beyond.

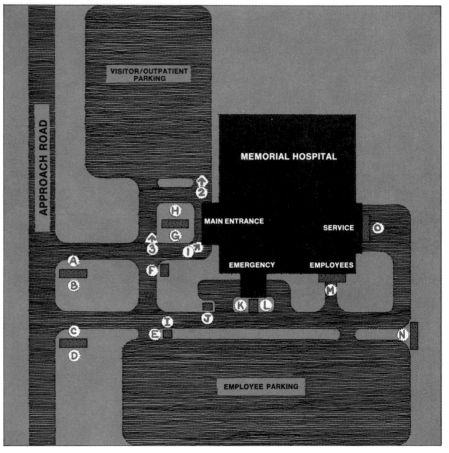

A.	Memorial Hospital ←Main Entrance ←Visitor Parking ↑Emergency ↑Service Entrance	**F.**	←Main Entrance ←Visitor Parking →Emergency	**N.**	←Service Entrance	
				O.	Service Entrance	
		G.	Memorial Hospital →Main Entrance ↑Visitor Parking	**1.**	Vehicular traffic should move in a counterclockwise direction past the main entrance.	
B.	Memorial Hospital →Main Entrance →Visitor Parking					
		H.	Memorial Hospital ←Main Entrance →Exit			
C.	Memorial Hospital ←Emergency ←Service Entrance			**2.**	Visitor parking should be beyond the drop-off point.	
		I.	←Emergency ←Service Entrance			
D.	Memorial Hospital →Emergency →Service Entrance ↑Main Entrance ↑Visitor Parking	**J.**	No Entry	**3.**	Traffic moving directly to the parking area should use a different route so as not to interfere with drop-off point.	
		K.	Emergency			
		L.	Emergency ↑Main Entrance ↑Exit			
E.	←Main Entrance ←Visitor Parking ↑Emergency ↑Service Entrance	**M.**	Employee Entrance			

When the approach road is heavily traveled, one service drive from which further distribution of traffic can be facilitated should be provided onto the site. In such a case, only the hospital identification sign is needed at the entrance drive. Secondary drives for the service, emergency department, and main entrances should follow the rules already outlined.

Vehicular traffic should move in a counterclockwise direction past the main entrance so that the entrance is on the passenger side of the vehicle. Visitor parking should be beyond the drop-off point. Traffic moving directly to the parking area should use a different route, so as not to interfere with traffic going to the drop-off point. A driver, having seen the main entrance, will know how to return to it once his car is parked, and this orientation will also help him find his car easily when he leaves the building.

When the approach road is heavily traveled, one service drive, from which distribution of traffic can be facilitated, should be provided. Vehicular traffic should move in a counterclockwise direction past the main entrance so that the entrance is on the passenger side of the vehicle.

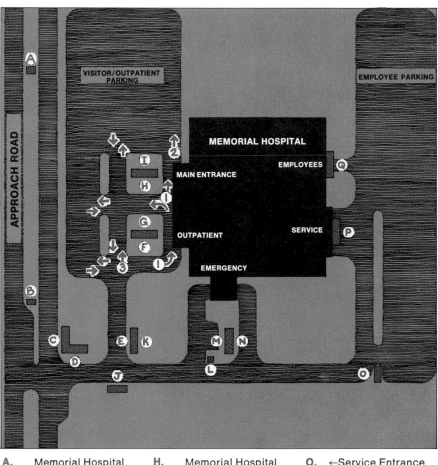

A. Memorial Hospital
Next Left

B. Memorial Hospital
←Emergency

C. Memorial Hospital
↑ Emergency

D. Memorial Hospital
→ Emergency

E. ←Outpatient Entrance
←Main Entrance
←Visitor Parking
↑ Emergency
↑ Service Entrance

F. Memorial Hospital
→Outpatient Entrance
↑ Main Entrance
↑ Visitor Parking

G. Memorial Hospital
←Outpatient Entrance
↑ Exit

H. Memorial Hospital
→Main Entrance
↑ Visitor Parking

I. Memorial Hospital
←Main Entrance
↑ Outpatient Entrance
↑ Exit

J. ←Emergency
←Service Entrance
→ Exit

K. →Outpatient Entrance
→Main Entrance
↑ Exit

L. No Entry

M. ←Emergency
↑ Service Entrance

N. →Emergency
↑ Main Entrance
↑ Exit

O. ←Service Entrance
↑ Employee Parking

P. Service Entrance

Q. Employee Entrance

1. Vehicular traffic should move in a counterclockwise direction past the entrances.

2. Visitor parking should be beyond the drop-off point.

3. Traffic moving directly to the parking area should use a different route so as not to interfere with drop-off point.

Outpatient and Emergency Drives

Separating visitor, outpatient, and emergency traffic patterns can be a problem, but it can be solved by a combination of design and indications that a separate access exists for each. If the emergency department entrance passes through a porte cochère, this and other appropriate architectural or landscape screening can imply restricted use. On the other hand, the main entrance can be identified by an open canopy, multiple entrance doors, and plantings—all of which emphasize the use of this entrance.

Accessibility is the key to appropriate outpatient traffic patterns, although outpatient movement will inevitably require directional or identifying signs. Design clues can help reinforce this movement. For example, outpatients can be discouraged from using the emergency department entrance if the emergency drive is separated from logical private vehicle movement patterns, is restricted in scale, has only a few spaces for short-term parking, and has no sidewalk.

Where a separate entrance for outpatients is provided, ideally it should be so located that a reception control point inside the building can oversee both this entrance and the emergency department entrance. This serves to facilitate staffing and permit separation of outpatients from emergency patients. When the outpatient department entrance is combined with the main entrance, less clear internal movement patterns result. Direction to the outpatient reception area is, of course, needed.

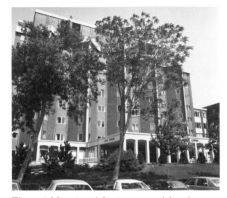

The architectural features and landscaping of this entrance connote this is a main entrance, not an emergency or an outpatient entrance.

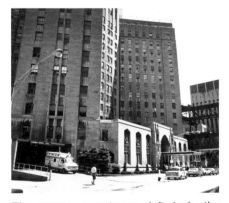

The emergency entrance, left, lacks the design clues of an open canopy and other architectural features of the main entrance, right.

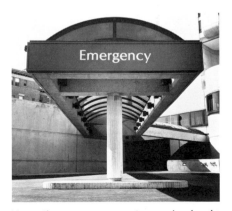

Here, the emergency entrance is clearly distinguishable by its identification and functional appearance.

Pedestrian Approaches

Pedestrian walkways should be provided between hospital parking areas and the main entrance. Such walkways can help keep visitors out of traffic lanes and direct them toward the right entrance and away from employee and emergency department entrances. A main entrance walkway that is wider than the secondary paths will guide visitors toward the entrance, as will the use of special materials, such as different paving, plantings, and other design elements.

Where patients and visitors arrive at the hospital by means of public transportation, signs may be needed at bus and subway stops to direct them to the hospital. Where possible, audible/tactile signs that are usable by the visually handicapped should also be provided. Signs are particularly important where the transportation stop is not immediately adjacent to the hospital. Approval of the size and the design of all signs and permission to post them must be obtained from the appropriate authorities.

The safety of intersections between public transportation stops and the hospital should also be considered. Are there stop signs or traffic lights? Are the curbs modified for wheelchair use? If such safety measures are lacking, the proper authorities can be petitioned to install them.

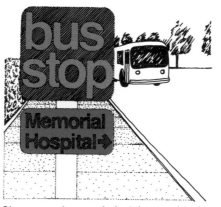

Signs may be needed at bus and subway stops to direct patients and visitors to the hospital.

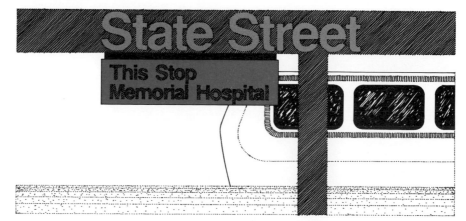

Situating Parking Areas

Careful planning of parking areas and the routes to them eliminates the need for many directional signs. Lack of a clear separation between entrance traffic and parking traffic is disorienting and results in a need for elaborate signs to direct traffic to the desired area. Signs can be used, however, to reinforce the identification of parking areas and to indicate limitations on their use· such as restrictions on the groups permitted (doctors, employees, visitors, handicapped, service) and on the amount of time allowed. The location of ramps for the handicapped should be clearly identified.

When employee parking is located beyond the service entrance, employees often use the service entrance drive. Employee parking should be located so that the most convenient access to the building is through the employees' entrance. It is often possible to locate a security checkpoint or purchasing office in such a way that it can oversee both the employee entrance and the service area.

For economy of construction and flexibility in assignment of parking spaces, particularly in a small hospital, it is often desirable to combine parking areas for visitors, medical staff, and employees. If this is done, identification and restriction signs are required for individual spaces or groups of spaces, and policing of the parking area may also be needed.

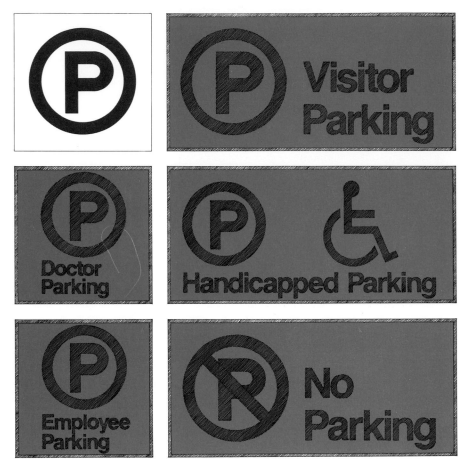

Identification and restriction signs for individual spaces or groups of spaces are necessary when parking areas for visitors, medical staff, and employees are combined.

Building entrances should be planned to relate to the parking area, whether or not parking for different categories of users is combined. When parking for different categories of users is combined, pedestrians coming from the parking area arrive at the hospital entrances primarily from one direction. If physical separation to identify entrances is not possible, explicit directional and identifying signs will be needed on the approach walks and at entrances. The information provided by the signs and the placement of them should follow the rules for signs at entrance drives from the approach road. In addition, "No Parking" signs should be posted at building entrances to avoid congestion.

When there is a multistoried parking structure, a number of additional elements must be considered. It is necessary for users to be able to locate the correct entrance to the hospital and return to their cars. Garage floor levels should be marked clearly and should be visible from every section. If the garage is served by an elevator, it is helpful to show the floor level at the elevator entrance. Sometimes the level number is applied directly to the outside of the elevator door. In a large parking structure, the floors should be subdivided into areas and even lanes, and these should be assigned identification letters or numbers. Signs that remind users to take note of the level and area numbers where their vehicles are parked are helpful.

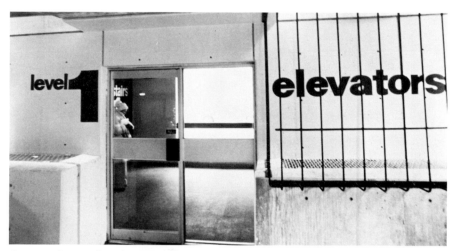

Garage elevator locations and floor numbers should be clearly marked.

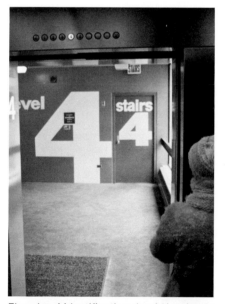

Floor-level identification should be clearly visible from elevators.

Because it is easy to become disoriented in a parking structure, it is important to have ample directional signs to guide users to the appropriate hospital entrance. If there is a single exit from the parking structure, it will suffice to have signs that guide the user to the exit, where specific directional signs can be placed. If there is more than one exit from the structure, signs pointing the way to the most appropriate exit for each hospital entrance must be placed throughout the structure. Some institutions located on large campuses provide simple maps showing how to reach each of the various buildings from the parking structure.

CHECKLIST FOR SITE PLANNING

When using this checklist, consider corrective measures that can be taken. Also, keep in mind that the sites should be barrier free, so that handicapped persons are not impeded.

1. Access roads
   Are highway signs at appropriate distances from the turnoffs?
   Are all access routes marked?
   Are directional signs placed at each decision point between the highway and the hospital?

2. Pedestrian access
   Can entrance(s) be seen from surface transportation stops?
   Are directional signs placed at each decision point along the path of pedestrian travel?
   Are there directional signs in mass transit stations?
   Are there stop signs or traffic lights where needed?
   Are there aids and cues for the visually handicapped?
   Are curbs modified for wheelchair use?
   Is wheelchair access clearly indicated?

3. Onsite traffic control
   Is the facility identified at site-entrance drive(s)?
   Is each building of a medical complex clearly identified?
   Is each special drive clearly identified?
       Service
       Emergency
       Parking lot(s)
       Other
   Are directions to reach other drives clearly indicated at each special drive turnoff?

4. Entrances
   Main entrance
   Is it visually a main entrance?
   Does vehicular traffic move counterclockwise past the en-
   trance? (Is the entrance on the passenger side of the vehicle?)
   Are there other entrances that are perceived as main
   entrances?
   Service entrance
   Is the service entrance clearly marked?
   Do unwanted vehicles enter?
   Is the loading dock clearly identified?
   Emergency department entrance
   Is the entrance appropriately identified in order to keep out all
   but emergency traffic?
   Is the entrance clearly differentiated from the outpatient de-
   partment entrance?
   Are directional signs placed at all site-access points and re-
   peated where necessary?
   Are ''No Parking'' signs placed appropriately?

5. Parking
   Are parking driveways distinct from approach driveways?
   Is the visitor parking entrance located beyond the main entrance
   drop-off?
   Is visitor parking located for ease of access to the main entrance?
   Is employee parking located near employee/service entrances?
   Is employee parking protected from unauthorized vehicles?
   Can staff enter the hospital from the parking lot without going
   through visitor/emergency/outpatient department areas?
   Are spaces reserved for the handicapped?

6. Onsite pedestrian traffic
   Are walkways and other design guides provided to direct traffic
   from visitor/outpatient department parking areas to appropriate
   entrances?
   Are crosswalks clearly marked?
   Are there aids and cues for the visually handicapped?
   Are curbs modified for wheelchair use?
   Is wheelchair access clearly indicated?

7. Parking structure pedestrian traffic
   Are floor levels clearly marked?
   Are areas or lanes marked?
   Are reminder signs placed at frequent intervals?
   Are directions to exit(s) visible from all parking areas?
   Are hospital entrances visible from the parking structure exit?
   If not, are there appropriate directional signs?

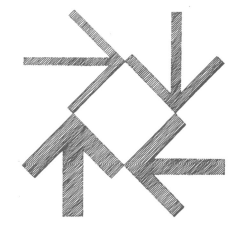

INTERIOR PLANNING

Many of the design principles that apply to exterior site planning apply equally to interior planning. When a hospital is planned on the basis of user categories rather than on the basis of departments or individual function, functional relationships are simplified and traffic movement is made easier. The six basic hospital user categories are public, outpatient, inpatient, paid and volunteer staffs, and service.

Good interior planning not only simplifies traffic movement within the building, but also helps make the building layout more comprehensible to the user and minimizes the need for directional signs. Grouping departments by functional relationships, providing orienting clues to the user, and carefully placing furnishings, wall treatments, and accessories can channel movement in desired patterns. For example, appropriate placement of furniture and plants can usually define a waiting area.

Planning in terms of large functional units at the outset can result in a less complicated pattern of general circulation and a clearer movement of secondary traffic. For example, consider the x-ray, laboratory, and physical therapy departments. Both outpatients and inpatients are likely to visit all three. When the departments are grouped, one basic movement pattern is required for inpatients and one for outpatients. When the departments are separated and dispersed, three outpatient and three inpatient patterns may be required—one pattern for each category of user of each service.

As another example, the medical library, the medical record department, and the physicians' lounge

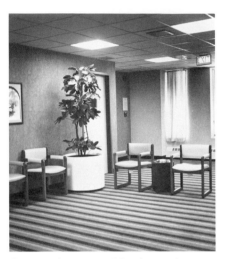

Careful placement of furniture, plants, or accessories can visually define a waiting area.

should all be convenient to the route to and from the physicians' parking lot. It may be difficult, if not impossible, to reorganize an existing building to improve access, circulation of traffic, and user orientation. However, in those instances where there are severe problems, consideration should be given to the cost effectiveness of relocating certain departments in order to develop more logical functional relationships.

Localization of site traffic and direction to specific entrances are the first steps in effectively communicating directions within the building. Therefore activities and facilities that are usually found on

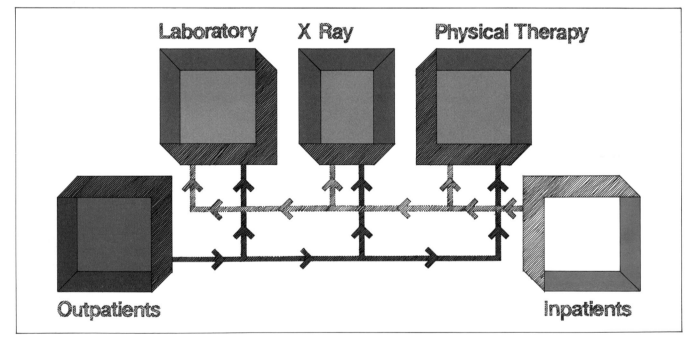

When both outpatients and inpatients are likely to visit the same group of departments, for example, laboratory, x-ray, and physical therapy, only one basic traffic pattern is required for each category of user.

the main floor should be located near the appropriate entrances and in the obvious movement patterns of the various groups of users. For example, the reception area, public elevators, waiting and admitting areas, cashier, and gift shop should be near the main entrance and readily visible. A glimpse of the outpatient waiting area or the reception point facilitates movement from the main entrance to this area. In public areas, people generally look for toilet rooms and telephones in subcorridors immediately adjacent to reception and waiting areas.

Emergency department reception and waiting areas should be immediately adjacent to the emergency department entrance. If possible, this area should be served by its own public telephones, toilet rooms, and vending machines to help eliminate unwanted traffic in other areas of the hospital. Such amenities should be located away from all work areas.

Orderly corridor schemes, based on careful functional planning, render buildings more understandable to the user. It is helpful to the user if he is able to orient himself to a known point. There are many ways in which this can be accomplished.

An atrium that is encountered by a person as he enters the building and reencountered as he moves through it helps him to maintain his bearings. Glazed walls that permit views of the outdoors, where recognizable structures or areas can be seen, can also help to orient the user. In certain long corridors, windows* overlooking internal activity can also help the user orient himself. This can be done effectively for staff members in the laundry, kitchen, central sterile supply, and mechanical plant areas. For visitors, a view of the cafeteria or pharmacy, for example, would be appropriate.

*The use of glass on interior corridor walls is limited by the National Fire Protection Association Life Safety Code no. 101.

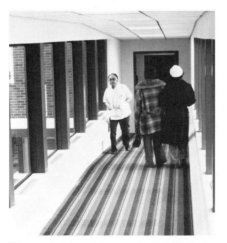

Views of the outdoors, where recognizable structures can be seen, help to orient the user.

Orientation can also be accomplished by the use of color (see chapter 5) or by the strategic placement of an arresting decorative piece, such as a painting, sculpture, wall hanging, mural, or the outsize letters, numbers, and designs known as supergraphics.

In short, any plan that will facilitate access to and progress through the building will help reduce the need for signs. Limiting the number of signs that will be needed saves money and serves to enhance the impact of those signs that *are* required.

When signs are required, they should be courteous. Particular attention should be given to signs at reception desks, cashiers' offices, and nurses' stations. All doors should be identified. Alarming signs, such as "Morgue" and "Autopsy," should be away from public view. "No Smoking" signs should be prominently displayed where appropriate. Aids for handicapped persons should be available and clearly marked.†

†See bibliography: *Accessibility—The Law and Reality*, 1974.

CHECKLIST FOR INTERIOR PLANNING

When using this checklist, consider corrective measures that can be taken. Also, keep in mind that all design should be barrier free, so that handicapped persons are not impeded.

1. Main entrance lobby
    Is the information/reception desk visible from the main entrance?
    Is the direction to the admitting office clearly indicated?
    Are public elevators visible? If public elevators are not visible, is direction given?
    Are amenities available and marked?
        Telephone
        Special telephones for hearing-handicapped persons and for wheelchair access
        Toilet rooms
        Coffee shop or other public eating facility
        Gift shop
        Vending machines
    Are routes to departments that are reached through the main lobby clearly indicated?
        Outpatient
        Radiology
        Cashier

2. Outpatient department
    Is the reception desk clearly marked?
    Does the reception desk have visual control of the waiting area?
    Can the user see the outpatient waiting room from the reception desk?
    Are amenities available and marked?
        Telephone
        Special telephones for hearing-handicapped persons and for wheelchair access
        Toilet rooms
        Public eating facilities
        Vending machines
    Are routes to the various clinical services clearly indicated?
    Is the first directional sign clearly visible from the reception desk?*
    If clinical services are some distance from the reception area:
        Are directions indicated at all intersections?*
        Are reinforcing signs placed at reasonable intervals?*
    Is the cashier's office clearly marked?*

*These items should be applied to each service offered in the outpatient department.

3. Emergency department
   Is the reception desk clearly marked?
   Is the reception desk placed so as to prevent unwanted traffic from passing?
   Does the reception desk have visual control of the waiting area?
   Are special offices marked?
      Security
      Press/police room
   Is the waiting room marked?
   Are amenities available and marked?
      Telephone
      Special telephones for hearing-handicapped persons and for wheelchair access
      Toilet rooms
      Vending machines

4. Patient floors
   Are floor numbers visible from elevators?
   Do directional signs at elevators indicate room number locations?
   Are there additional directional signs at all corridor intersections?
   Are there directional signs to lounge areas?
   Are all doors clearly marked?
      Patient rooms
      Utility closets
      Staff facilities
      Toilet rooms
      Conference rooms
      Meeting rooms
      Other
   Do room numbers follow a discernible pattern?
   Are telephone numbers coordinated with room numbers?
   Is coordination desirable?

5. All areas
   Are all exits clearly marked?
   Are emergency instructions marked?
      Fire
      Disaster
   Are fire alarm systems marked?
      Pull stations
      Fire extinguisher locations for classes A, B, and C
   Are utility hookups marked?
      Air
      Electric
      Oxygen
      Vacuum
      Other
   Are smoking areas clearly marked?

4

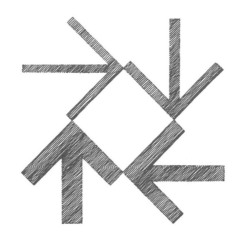

DATA COLLECTION

Developing a signs and graphics system takes considerable time, and eventually it will require the services of many persons in addition to the architect and the landscape architect, who already have been mentioned. Hospital consultants, graphic designers, and others will be called in for advice at the appropriate time. The accompanying chart shows the relationship between the in-house sign committee and outside consultants.

However, depending on the relative availability of money and personnel, much of the data gathering and analysis can be done either in-house by a sign committee or outside by a consultant. The sign committee might consist of representatives of the administration; nursing and ambulatory services; and the purchasing, engineering, and maintenance departments. Others might be from public relations, ancillary services, and the business office.

The key person is the sign committee coordinator, who is chiefly responsible for controlling the work. The coordinator works directly with outside professionals and in-house staff who are engaged in the making, installing, or buying of the signs and graphics.

Whoever does the actual work, development of the system can take a year or more from idea to completion. Up to four months should be allowed for gathering and analyzing information, two months for preparing specifications and taking bids from manufacturers, and up to six months for fabricating and installing the signs.

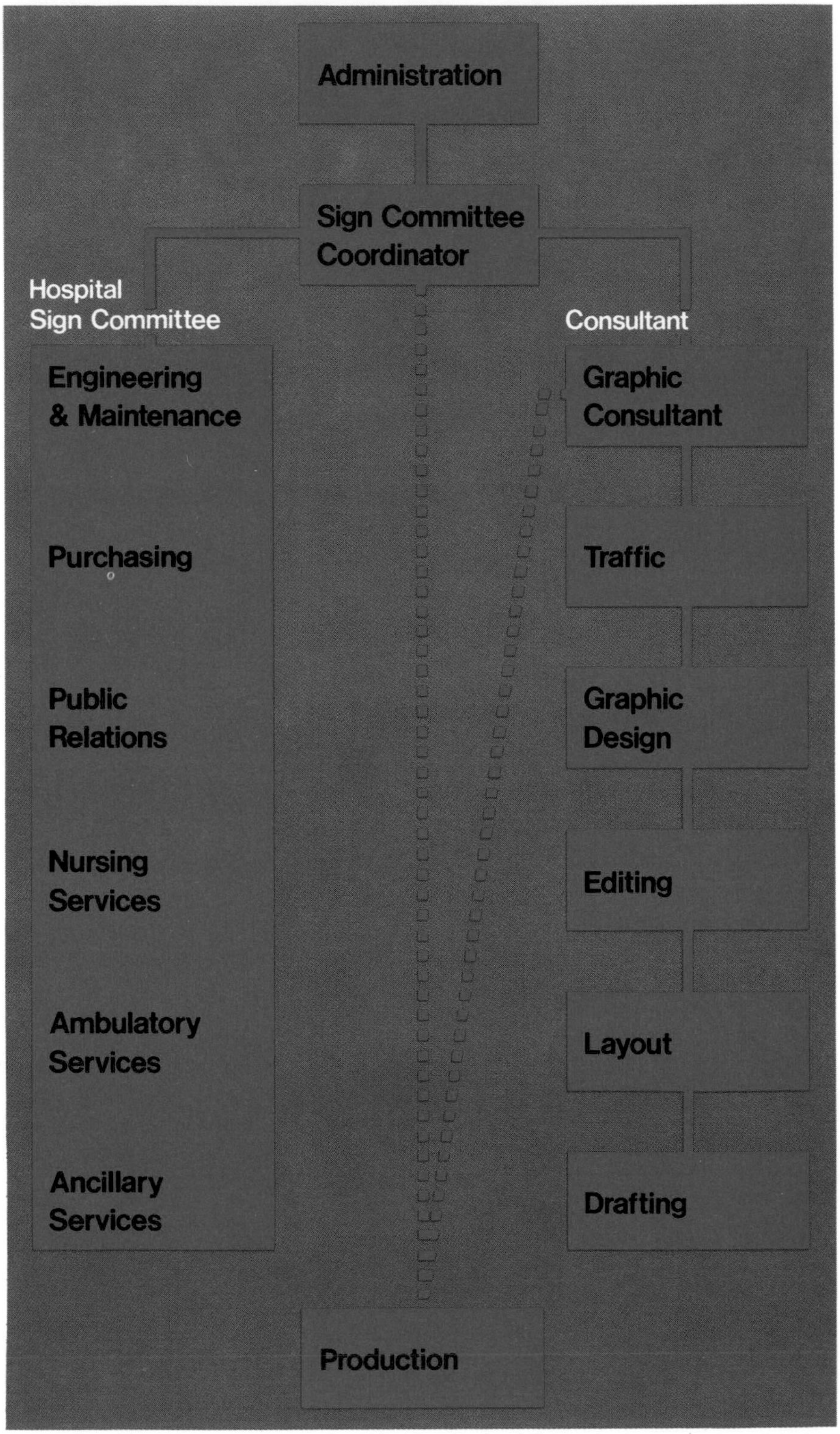

Administration

Sign Committee
Coordinator

Hospital
Sign Committee

Engineering
& Maintenance

Purchasing

Public
Relations

Nursing
Services

Ambulatory
Services

Ancillary
Services

Consultant

Graphic
Consultant

Traffic

Graphic
Design

Editing

Layout

Drafting

Production

The development of a signs and graphics system requires the time and services of many persons.

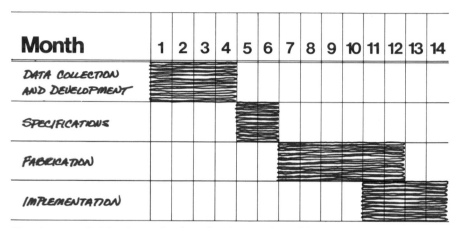

Month	1	2	3	4	5	6	7	8	9	10	11	12	13	14
DATA COLLECTION AND DEVELOPMENT	■	■	■	■										
SPECIFICATIONS					■	■								
FABRICATION							■	■	■	■	■	■		
IMPLEMENTATION											■	■	■	■

The steps needed for the realization of a signs and graphics system can take a year or more.

Determining Uses and Conditions

The first step in the development of a signs and graphics system is data collection, a process of charting the existing situation and the needs of the users and then comparing one against the other. The checklists in this book help accomplish this step.

The first phase of data collection is the determination of the groups of users and their needs. For each user group, certain characteristics must be considered: age, physical capacity, and comprehension. For patients, diagnosis also must be considered. Patients and visitors may be any age from the very young to the elderly; staff members are usually active adults; service personnel may range from a young adult to the elderly. Patients, visitors, and staff may have physical, visual, or aural handicaps, and all groups may have mental handicaps or use primarily a foreign language.

Each of these characteristics must be evaluated in terms of light, medium, and heavy traffic volume and whether the traffic flow is one way or multidirectional. Analysis of these factors will help to determine the types and numbers of signs required.

The special requirements of the various groups of users differ from one hospital to another and in each department and on different floors. For example, if the hospital is located in a population center where there are many non-English-speaking residents, bilingual signs should be considered for at least those areas where visitors and unescorted patients are expected to find their way unaided. If bilingual signs are determined to be necessary, it is reasonable to assume that there should also be bilingual personnel—paid or volunteer—available at the reception and information desks.

The needs of persons with various kinds of physical handicaps must also be considered. For example, wheelchair access should be clearly indicated. For the vis-

ually handicapped, Occupational Safety and Health Administration requirements call for knurled doorknobs at all exits to stairwells. Knurling, that is, roughing up the surface of the handle or engraving a symbol or braille language on it, warns the individual not to pass through that doorway or enter the area. On existing wood handles, knurling is easily done in-house. For metal handles, rubber disks bearing an embossed warning are available and are easily attached. Other special aids such as braille floor numbers in elevators may

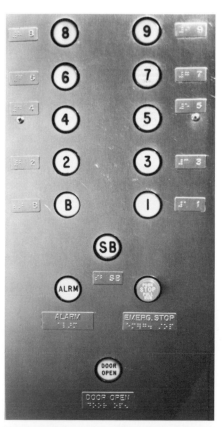

Floor numbers in elevators should be indicated in braille as well as in the usual manner.

also be needed. Indeed, local codes may require such special information aids, and some jurisdictions require raised lettering and numbering for certain types of signs and dictate their placement.

The next phase of data collection is the preparation of a specific statement of existing conditions within the hospital and on the site. The person responsible for the statement should walk outside and through the hospital, imagining he is unfamiliar with the layout and location of various departments, and judge for himself whether or not a person visiting the hospital for the first time would be able to find his way around with minimal help. He should pick a starting point, perhaps the main lobby, and go to a particular destination, for example, the coffee shop, by using only the available sources of information, not his prior knowledge. He should do this for several destinations and from different points of origin and make notes of his experiences.

It is essential to enlist the cooperation of staff members, particularly nurses, in the data collection phase, because they are familiar with the kinds of questions patients and visitors ask and the kinds of directional help most frequently needed. One way to ensure cooperation is to be sure that staff members understand the ultimate benefit of a good signs and graphics system not only to patients and visitors, but to themselves. A proposal for a system could be put on the agenda for a staff meeting at which a representative of the administration could explain the plan to develop a new system and its benefits. The administration could also request help in identifying trouble spots and those places where confusion frequently occurs.

All staff members who come in frequent direct contact with patients and visitors should be asked to keep an informal record showing how many requests for directions they answer, what directions are asked for, and who asked the questions—patients, visitors, or employees. A definite date should be set for reporting back this information; two weeks is probably enough.

Information provided by the staff, answers to the checklist questions, and personal observations should round out the picture of existing conditions. The next step is to plot this picture on site and floor plans of the hospital.

Plotting the Information

Floor plans should reflect present use of rooms and show any alterations made since the hospital was built. If the plans are more complex than necessary for data-gathering purposes, as is usually true of blueprints, they should be redrawn in simpler form, showing only room outlines, doors, elevators, corridors, and so forth. The building engineer can probably accomplish this.

Drawings should indicate the various departments, such as outpatient, emergency, and radiology; reception and admitting areas; and at least one typical nursing floor, showing the relationships of patient rooms, elevators, waiting areas, nurses' stations, and so forth. All floor plans should be drawn to the same scale.

A hospital may have special needs that will require drawings different from those illustrated here. The illustrations are examples only, and the actual numbers and types of drawings should be determined by the requirements of the particular facility.

Several transparent sheets will be needed to use as overlays on the plans. These can be made of inexpensive tracing paper. Acetate sheets can also be used. Although the acetate is more expensive, it is also more durable. It can be wiped clean if desired, so that changes can be made easily. Plans can be drawn freehand with a felt-tip marker. All these supplies are available at art supply stores.

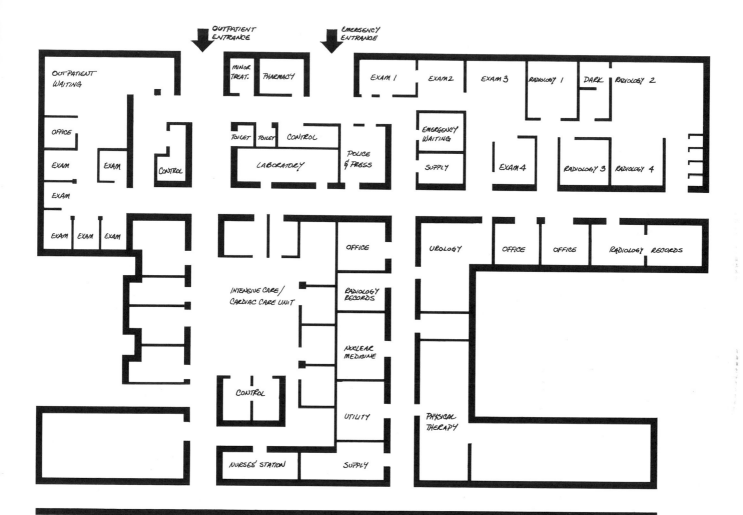

Complex plans should be redrawn to show only room outlines, doors, elevators, corridors, and other major plan elements, and spaces should be identified.

The first overlay is placed over the simplified floor plan, and the main departments are outlined. Next, on the same overlay, each outlined area, including the corridors, is blocked out.

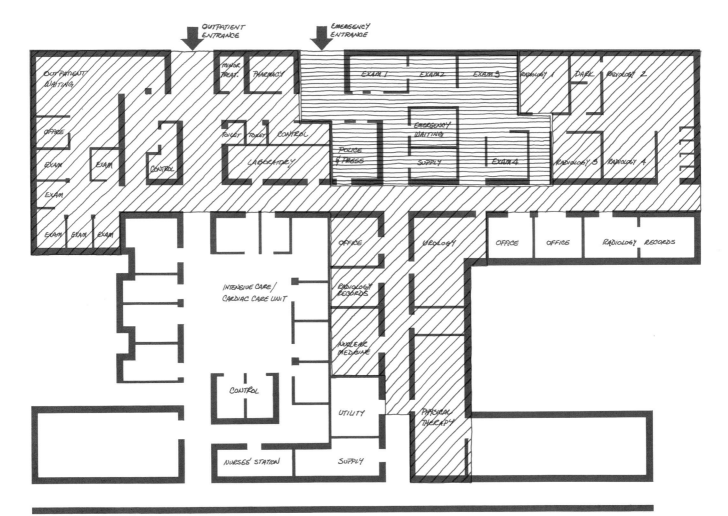

An overlay is placed on the simplified plan, and the main departments are blocked out according to appropriate users.

Next, on a second overlay, the desirable traffic patterns for various types of users are indicated. Only staff should be in some areas; in others, staff and patients; and elsewhere, all users may be welcome. Different-colored markers or tapes can be used to indicate these patterns. For example, red can be used for emergency traffic and blue for outpatient traffic.

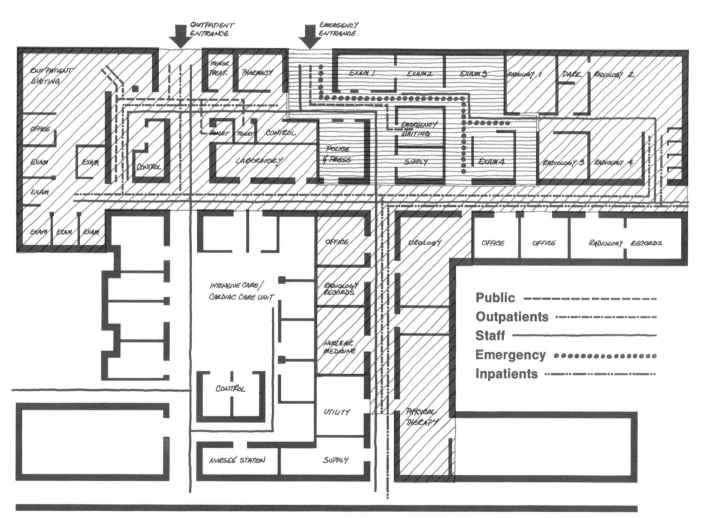

The desirable traffic patterns are then marked on a second overlay.

On a third overlay, the data are plotted by marking the trouble spots identified by the staff. For example, if many individuals are reported as having trouble finding the pharmacy, the corridor and entrance to that area should be marked. Or, if visitors are using the employee or the emergency entrance, this should be shown. Clusters of trouble spots that appear outside desired traffic pat-terns probably identify areas where the present information system is inadequate. It is also helpful to indi-cate the place where questions are asked. If a technician working in a laboratory that is located beyond the outpatient x-ray department is frequently asked for directions to the x-ray department, this is an indication that existing signs—di-rectional, informational, or both—are not clear.

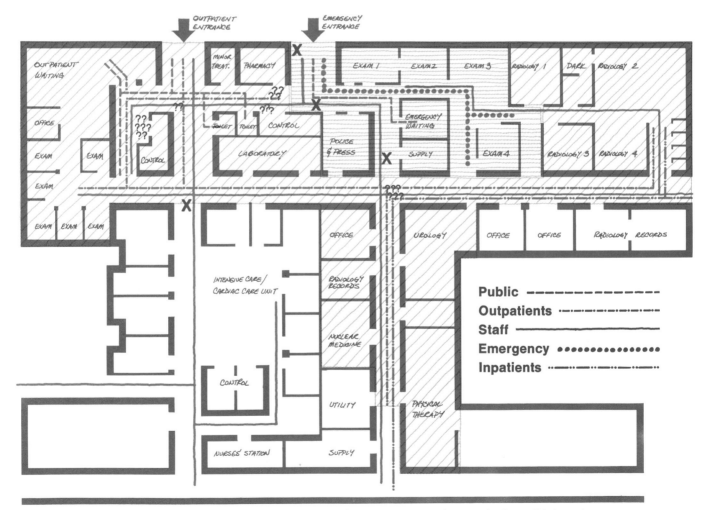

Trouble spots where many patients or visitors ask for information or are unwanted are marked on a third overlay.

Locations at which changes are required are marked on the final overlay. Trouble spots plotted on the previous overlay will be visible. The kinds of changes that ultimately will be made will depend upon the circumstances. For example, finding the pharmacy might be made easier by the addition of a sign, whereas keeping unwanted persons out of the intensive care unit might require the installation of a door.

When plotting trouble spots and desirable traffic patterns, the site should not be overlooked. Reports of unauthorized vehicles using a doctors' parking area may reflect inadequate visitors' parking; on the other hand, they may indicate that the entrance to the visitors' parking area is not clearly marked.

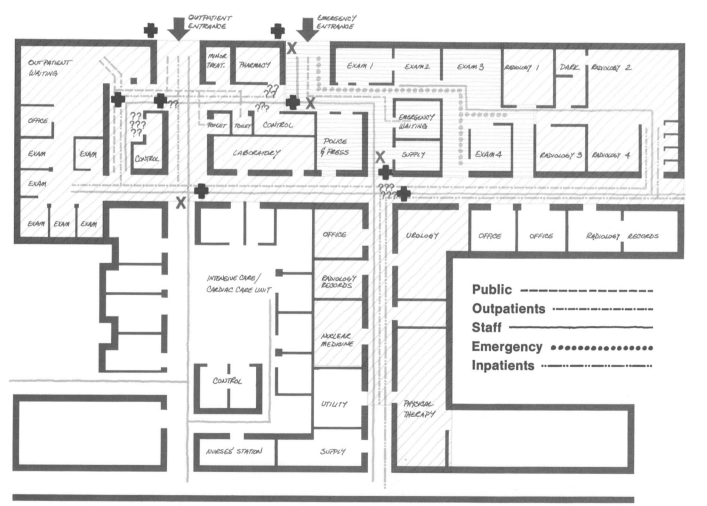

On the final overlay, points where change is needed are plotted. Changes may include new or different information or a traffic barrier such as a door.

Determining the Signs You Need

From this set of plans and overlays, the required directional signs or other forms of orientation and information can be determined. Orientation can be provided in a number of ways. As described in chapter 2, views to the outdoors can be useful in providing orientation and reassurance. Color coding of areas, departments, wings, or floors can be a part of the overall information system. However, it is not desirable to use permanent or semipermanent color coding to identify departments or functions that might later be moved to another location. If the floor layout is not too complex, a large "you are here" diagram, strategically located, can aid orientation and take the place of a forest of confusing signs.

Signs should be located at every point where the user has a choice of direction: at corridor intersections, turnings, stairs, and so forth. In some situations, reinforcing signs may be needed at intervals even when a decision is not required. In a long corridor, for example, a directional sign repeated at intervals can reassure the newcomer that he has not passed the place he is looking for. If the route to a particular department is long or complicated, it may be desirable to have a reinforcing directional sign always in view. In addition, floor numbers should be indicated on interior stairwell doors and on walls opposite elevator doors.

Once trouble areas have been identified and the reasons for problems have been made clear, a list should be made, by department, of all the rooms and spaces that need to be identified. Usually, every door should bear some identification, because unidentified doors tend to attract intruders. A lost visitor is less liable to blunder into a linen room that is clearly marked "Linen Room" than one with a numbered or unmarked door. Various types of identification are needed for different purposes. For example, each linen room and janitor's closet needs to be identified for the housekeeping and engineering personnel, but these spaces do not need to be part of the room numbering scheme used by visitors. The list of rooms and spaces eventually will be used to determine the number of identifying signs and/or numbers required. Rooms with more than one door will require more than one sign, and this must be so noted on the list.

A person should then be assigned to tour the hospital and copy the messages on each existing sign. Inconsistencies in terminology, even in such simple messages as "Ladies" and "Women," are likely to be observed. This list should include notations of all temporary signs, such as "Oxygen in Use," "Isolation," and other signs that may be used intermittently for patient care. It should also make note of such things as memorial plaques and bulletin boards, which are not always thought of as signs. And it should include movable, or sliding panel, signs that indicate vacant or occupied conference rooms, tub rooms, and other facilities.

Once the signs that will be needed have been determined, it is time to develop a uniform vocabulary for signs.

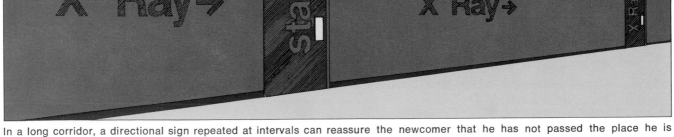

In a long corridor, a directional sign repeated at intervals can reassure the newcomer that he has not passed the place he is looking for.

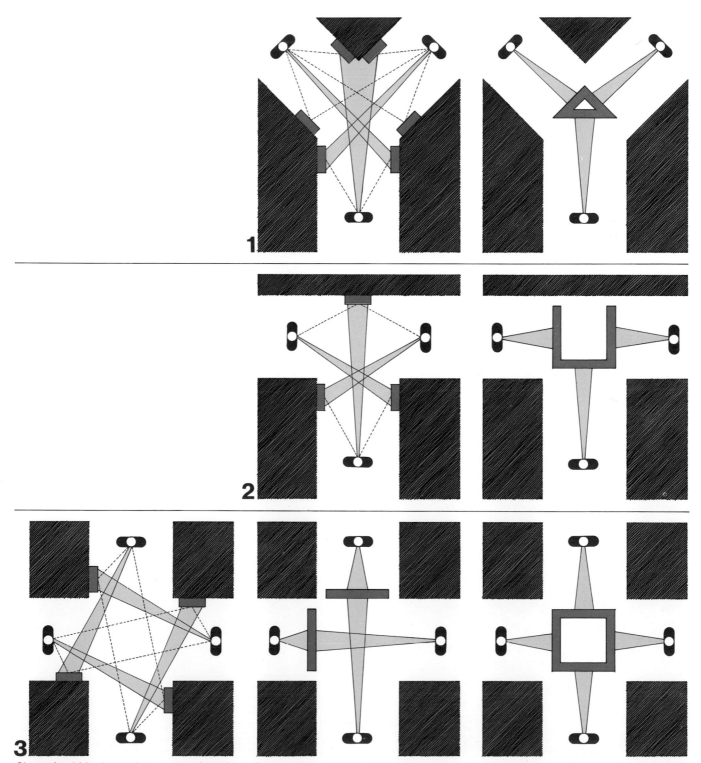

Signs should be located at every point where the user has a choice of direction. At corridor intersections, signs can be placed as illustrated. 1, Y intersections; 2, T intersections; 3, cross intersections.

CHECKLIST FOR DATA COLLECTION

1. Who are the users:
   Inpatients?
   Outpatients?
   Professional staff?
   Employees?
   Visitors?
   Emergency department patients?
   Delivery people?
   Other?

2. What *special* needs do users have:
   Bilingual signs?
   Aids for the visually handicapped?
   Wheelchair access?
   Other?

3. What kinds of room and building numbering are required:
   Patient rooms?
   Outpatient department rooms?
   Room inventory?
   Buildings?
   Building wings?

4. What kinds of interior and exterior signs will be included:
   Direction?
   Identification?
   Numbering?
   Memorial plaques?
   Highway and road signs?
   Warning?
   Prohibitory?
   Explanatory?
   Temporary?

5

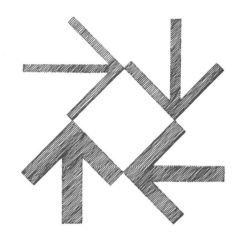

CHOOSING MESSAGES AND MEDIA

An information system consists not only of words, written and spoken, but also of graphic elements. Symbols, pictures, colors, and supergraphics can all play a part in directing users to and through the hospital.

Terminology

Because words will undoubtedly form the largest part of any system, and because much information is too abstract or too complex to be conveyed entirely by pictures, words will be considered first.

The process of developing a new signs and graphics system provides a good opportunity for thinking about standardized nomenclature for use throughout the hospital. Phasing out certain words in common hospital use that may have developed negative connotations should also be considered. For example, *continuing care* or *long-term care* can be substituted for chronic care and *services* can be substituted for clinic. Certain technical or medical terms can be changed into layman's language. Signs for the handicapped should be incorporated into the system. It is also a good time to review staff titles and administrative terminology for consistency and clarity.

Traditionally, hospital departments have been identified by means of medical terminology that can be easily understood only by doctors and other hospital personnel. This can be a serious problem, particularly for outpatients, who often must go unescorted to other departments. Also, the unnecessary labeling of spaces with medical terminology can create problems for support personnel, who often are volunteers. Their duties can take them to almost any part of the hospital, but their visits to any one location may be too infrequent for them to become familiar with hospital terminology and layout.

The trend, particularly in outpatient areas, seems to be toward the use of nontechnical layman's language in place of medical terminology—for example, eye care rather than ophthalmology. It is important to note, however, that sometimes these usages can cause more confusion than they eliminate. *Child care,* for example, could mean pediatrics, a nursery, or playroom facilities for the children of outpatients or visitors.

For certain medical departments or specialties there just do not seem to be any plain-language equivalents. But when such equivalents exist and their use is appropiate, they can help make communication easier.

Thinking through the matter of terminology may show that not all members of the staff use the same terms to refer to the same hospital areas and functions and that words on existing signs are far from uniform. Some of the various designations for toilet rooms have already been referred to in the preceding chapter. Functional areas of the hospital may likewise be referred to in a variety of ways. For example, one employee may refer to central sterile supply, and another may speak of central processing and delivery. This becomes even more confusing when the departments are referred to by their initials, CSS and CPD, as they frequently are in conversation.

A standard nomenclature can be developed from the list of messages compiled (see chapter 4). It is essential that the list be complete and that every variation in wording be included. Words and phrases should be grouped together according to the message they convey; for example, all signs that say, in one way or another, toilet room: women, ladies, women patients, women employees, ladies lounge, powder room; men, gentlemen, men patients, men employees. Another set might be those signs that refer to eating facilities: cafeteria, coffee shop, vending machines, employee cafeteria, doctors' dining room, snack shop, lunchroom. A third set could refer to outpatient medical services.

When all the words are grouped, each group should be looked at with the aim of eliminating unnecessary synonyms. It is probably necessary to differentiate between patients' and visitors' toilets, but not necessary to distinguish men from gentlemen. Remember that cutting down on word variety also means eliminating some expense.

Signs are classified in four broad categories:

Movement
- Orientation. You are *here.*
- Direction. You wish to go *there* and you get *there* this way.

Information
- Positive. You *may* act.
- Negative. You *may not* act.

Advisory or cautionary
- Attention is needed.

Identification
- You have *arrived* at your destination.

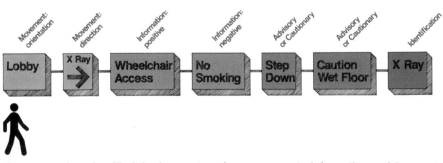

Signs can be classified in four categories: movement, information, advisory or cautionary, and identification.

Symbols and Pictographs

Words can frequently be supplemented, if not replaced, by graphics. For communication purposes these usually take the forms of symbols and pictographs. Although a distinction can be made between symbols and pictographs, it frequently becomes blurred. A pictograph is a picture that represents an idea literally—a figure in a wheelchair represents the physically handicapped. A symbol is a picture of something that is generally understood and accepted as representing an abstract concept—a caduceus symbolizes the art of healing, which is personified in the physician. The arrow, used for indicating direction, is one of the oldest and most universally understood symbols. In red on a white ground, the Greek cross, with arms of equal length, has come to be accepted as a symbol for emergency aid and is thus often used as a quick means of identifying medical equipment or supplies.

The letters of our alphabet also are symbols in that, alone or in combination, they represent ideas. The letters T-R-E-E do not resemble the shape of a tree. If they did, they would be a pictograph. This illustrates another difference between symbols and pictographs. A pictograph should immediately convey information to anyone who understands the cultural environment; the meaning of a symbol must be learned.

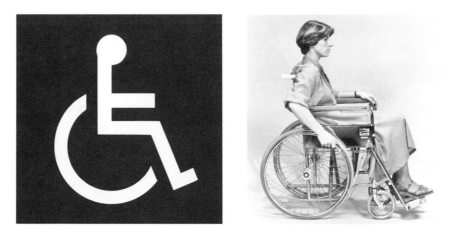

A pictograph is a representation of an object.

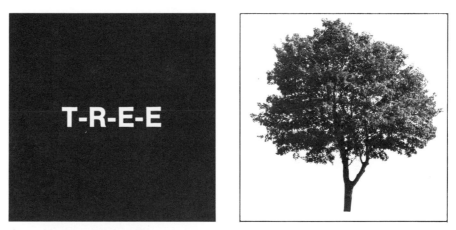

A word is a symbol that expresses an idea or represents an object.

A symbol can be used in place of words, and its meaning must be learned.

Familiarity with the culture is important. Cultural differences can have a major effect on an individual's ability to comprehend the intended meaning of symbols and pictographs. For example, a stork carrying a bundle in a diaper is occasionally used in hospitals to indicate the entrance to the labor-delivery suite. Whereas the stork is still enough a part of the Western culture to have some meaning in this context, it is not universally understood.

Several systems of symbols and pictographs have been developed or adapted specifically for hospitals and can be very helpful, especially when used in combination with words that are necessarily technical or have no plain-language equivalents. These graphic devices can serve other purposes in addition to simple communication. They can amuse, divert, reassure, or add to the decorative scheme.

Pictographs and symbols can also modify behavior in ways that words alone often cannot. This can be true in situations where prohibitions are necessary—for example, ''No Smoking.'' When pictographs are used in such situations, the prohibition may be met with less hostility (if hostility can be measured in terms of disobedience or even vandalism).

IN THE MUSEUM...
PLEASE... MUSE, CONVERSE, SMOKE, STUDY, STROLL, TOUCH, ENJOY, LITTER, RELAX, EAT, LOOK, LEARN; TAKE NOTES WITH PEN, PENCIL...

Photo: Courtesy Hirschhorn Museum and Sculpture Garden, Washington, DC.
Words and symbols can present a prohibition in a positive, pleasant manner, as is demonstrated by this sign.

Many pictographs commonly used in hospitals and other public places employ the red diagonal bar in a circle to indicate a prohibition. The diagonal bar has long been used in Europe and is becoming common in the United States. Thus, a smoldering cigarette in a circle, with a diagonal slash, means ''No Smoking,'' and just about everybody understands.

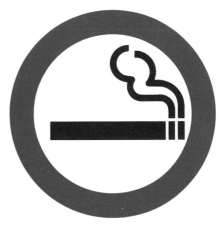

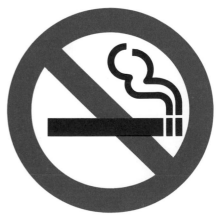

Just about everybody understands that a red diagonal bar across a circle is a prohibitory sign.

Standardization of symbols and pictographs does not seem to be likely in the immediate future. Even what is called the international system is not universal. Nevertheless, the content, if not the form, of many symbols and pictographs can be stated. Generally accepted examples of content are described in the accompanying table.

Most systems of pictographs are copyrighted by their designers and may not be used without permission.

A system of special symbols required to be used in hospitals has been developed by the National Fire Protection Association for the identification of degrees of health hazard, flammability, and reactivity (instability) of various types of stored materials. This information is presented in a color-coded spatial diagram of the three hazards, each hazard numerically indicated according to its degree of severity.* These signs can be applied on storage or processing tanks or on large pipelines that transport hazardous materials.

The temptation to "overgraphic" the system should be resisted. If there is any chance that a symbol or pictograph will confuse rather than clarify, that it might lead the user to a conclusion other than the one intended, then words should be used.

The matter of highway signs should be discussed with local and/or state highway authorities. For example, although the white capital H on a blue background is the official U.S. Department of Transportation highway sign and the internationally accepted sign meaning hospital, is the H symbol together with a directional arrow to designate the location of a hospital sufficient? Or should other information also appear, such as the hospital name where several hospitals are located in a particular area? Should "Trauma Center" be indicated if the hospital is so designated?

The U.S. Department of Transportation's National Highway Traffic Safety Administration has adopted the "star of life" symbol for use on all emergency medical care vehicles. The blue symbol depicts the staff of Aesculapius.

Bath	Tub in elevation
Coffee shop	Cup and saucer
Coronary care/ cardiac care	Valentine heart shape
Dental care	Tooth shape, with crown and roots
Emergency	Blue "star of life" with the staff of Aesculapius, or a red Greek cross on a white field
Ear, nose, and throat care	Stylized human profile, with three dots representing ear, nose, throat
Eye care/ophthalmology	Eye shape
Handicapped access	Wheelchair in elevation
Hematology/blood donors	Red drop with Greek cross inside
Laboratory	Microscope in elevation
Men's toilet room	Male figure with legs apart and arms in down position
Nursery	Three stylized infants (circle with features representing head, swaddled body)
Oxygen	Oxygen bottle in elevation, or green and white bottle in yellow triangle (Occupational Safety and Health Administration)
Parking	Uppercase P
Pharmacy	Uppercase R with slash through tail, or mortar and pestle
Podiatry	Right foot print
Prohibitions:	
No smoking	Cigarette, with smoke, in red circle with red diagonal slash
No parking	P in red circle with diagonal slash
No entry	Red disk with broad white horizontal bar across center
Restaurant	Vertical knife and fork
Shower	Shower head with dots representing water
Stairway	Staircase, side view, with person in elevation
Telephone	Telephone handset in elevation
Urology	Two kidney shapes
Women's toilet room	Female figure with legs together and arms in down position
X ray/radiology	Male figure with trunk and legs within a rectangle representing film

---

*See bibliography: National Fire Protection Association. *National Fire Codes.*

Color

The following suggestions about the use of color pertain to signs and directional graphics and are not intended as restrictions on the use of color as a design element in the hospital. In Western culture, certain colors have particular connotations and therefore have been used for signs in particular contexts.

The color red often connotes blood or fire and, by extension, danger. Red on signs should therefore be reserved to indicate emergency, prohibition, and warning. In addition to the previously noted red diagonal bar in a circle, fire extinguishers and exit signs are red, as is the white-barred red disk indicating no entry. Yellow is traditionally used where caution is required, because of its particular visibility and attention-getting qualities. The caution sign is triangular in shape and can warn of slippery floors or bad traffic conditions. Green generally indicates permission to go. Blue denotes available information and services.

The Occupational Safety and Health Administration (OSHA) has probably done more than any other agency in the United States to make uniform the use of color as a device for transmitting information in institutions. OSHA regulations apply to hospitals as places of work and must be adhered to in the development of the hospital signs and graphics system. Briefly, OSHA rules stipulate red for firefighting equipment, containers for flammable or otherwise dangerous substances, elevator "stop" buttons, and electrical switches; green for safety and first-aid equipment; yellow for cau-

tion; and magenta for radiation hazards. The radiation symbol, a magenta trefoil shape on a yellow ground, is an example of the combination of two messages, "radiation" and "caution," and is an OSHA requirement.

Apart from the traditional symbolic uses of color, color is often used to differentiate wings, floors, or buildings of a hospital complex. A color-coding scheme carried out completely and logically throughout the institution can be useful in helping the visitor sort out a multiplicity of departments, areas, and services. Inexpensive and easily changed color coding for the purpose of orientation can be achieved with paint on key walls, such as those opposite elevators or at corridor turns or ends. It can be risky, however, to try to create many color-coded "pathways" to various departments within the hospital, because departmental locations are frequently changed. Pathways indicated by colored carpeting, flooring, or painted stripes would then have to be changed as well—an onerous and probably expensive process.

Factors that affect the perception of colors include the lighting conditions under which they are seen, sources of the light, and the colors that surround them. Perception of internally illuminated signs is somewhat different from that of opaque colors viewed under ambient lighting. For example, from a distance it is difficult or impossible to differentiate between small blue and green light sources (as in illuminated signs) and between orange and yellow ones. Red and green (or blue) light sources are easiest to recog-

nize, and yellow (or orange) sources are the most difficult. White light sources fall between these two extremes.

When seen under similar light conditions, opaque colors also have different qualities. Opaque yellow is the most visible and luminous, orange and red-orange offer maximum attention value, and blue is likely to be indistinct.

Legible color combinations, ranging from the most to the least legible, are black on white, black on yellow, green on white, white on green, red on white, and white on blue. Combinations of pure red and green or red and blue are not satisfactory.

Mock-up signs using painted cardboard and press-on lettering can be made in order to test the relative legibility of various color combinations and letter sizes under actual conditions of use. Mock-ups will also help to determine the optimum height for placing wall-mounted signs. As an alternative to homemade mock-ups, sign manufacturers may be willing to supply samples in the actual sizes and materials to be used.

Use of mock-ups and samples can also help in developing a sign system that will be harmonious with the colors of wall and trim finishes and other design elements. For example, sign panels of a particular color can seem like a good idea until that color is tested against a wall or door that has been painted a similar or clashing color, or under lights that change its tone. Unless signs can be matched to specified wall paint colors, it is best to use accent colors for the signs.

6

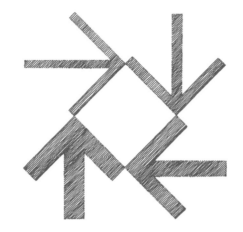

CHOOSING SIGNS

After having decided what messages should be conveyed through what words, symbols, pictographs, and colors, the signs themselves should be considered. In order for signs to be quickly understandable, they must be legible. Sign legibility is achieved by careful selection of letter style, design, size, color, contrast, spacing, and placement.

A sign system will have greater overall visual authority and clarity if consistency is maintained in typeface style, margins, letter spacing, placement, and, if possible, color within each category of sign.

The following terms and explanations facilitate communication between the administrator and the designer or the manufacturer. These terms are used by graphic designers, sign manufacturers, and suppliers of lettering and sign-making equipment to describe the common physical characteristics of letters. Many reference works are available for additional technical information (see bibliography, page 63).

Ascender:
The part of a lowercase letter that extends to about the height of the capital letter, such as the upper sections of the letters *b, d, f,* and *k.*

Baseline:
An imaginary line on which align the bottoms of capital and/or lowercase letters without descenders.

Copy:
The text of the material to be reproduced; the manuscript.

Descender:
The portion of a lowercase letter that descends below the baseline of the letter, as in the letters *g, j, p, q,* and *y.*

Face:
See **Typeface**

Font:
A complete assortment of types of one typeface and size, including capitals, small capitals, lowercase letters, and numerals and punctuation.

Italic:
A style of type in which the letters slant to the right, as differentiated from the upright roman style, which is customarily used for books and newspapers. Italic is often used for emphasis and is indicated on copy by underlining.

Line space:
The vertical distance occupied by one line of type measured baseline to baseline of lines above and below.

Point:
The basic unit of measurement in printing; there are approximately 72 points to one inch.

Roman:
Upright letters and numbers, which are the standard style of print used in books and newspapers. The designation stems from the capital forms, which are modeled on ancient Roman inscriptions and are distinct from the italic style.

Sans serif:
Any typeface without serifs, or finishing lines, on the ends of strokes and without pronounced variation in thickness of the stroke.

Serif:
A finishing line or stroke crossing or projecting from the end of a main line or stroke of a letter.

This is a roman typeface.

This is an italic typeface.

This is a sans serif typeface.

This is a serif typeface.

Typeface:
The design of the type; for example, Helvetica typeface.

X-cap height:
The height of the capital letter in a particular typeface.

Lowercase x-height:
The distance between the top and the bottom of a printed letter, such as *x, a, c,* and *w,* without an ascender or descender; also the corresponding dimension in the type from which such letters are printed.

Typeface

Because the user must be able to distinguish signs and register their messages quickly, it is essential that the typeface chosen for them be easily legible.

Typefaces for signs should be simple and uncluttered; decorative typefaces are better left for the printed page, where the reader has time to absorb the content more leisurely. Although there appears to be a trend toward the use of all lowercase letters in signs, most persons find it easier and quicker to understand signs that use a combination of capital and lowercase letters. This is because the reader can recognize word shapes from distances at which individual letters cannot be distinguished.

For signs, sans serif typefaces are generally considered more readable than serif faces. Of the sans serif faces, Helvetica is becoming increasingly popular and is available in many materials, including cutout and press-on letters, which are an advantage if the system is to include temporary signs or signs made in-house. Another advantage of Helvetica is that many sign fabricators and manu-

This is Helvetica
roman type.
It is a sans serif
typeface.

*This is Helvetica
italic type.
It is a sans serif
typeface.*

This is
Century Schoolbook
roman type.
It is a serif
typeface.

*This is
Century Schoolbook
italic type.
It is a serif
typeface.*

facturers carry stock signs in this typeface. These stock signs can often be incorporated into custom-designed sign systems at a cost savings. However, other equally legible and satisfactory typefaces are available, including some with serifs.

Typefaces often are available in three weights—light, medium, and bold—and also in condensed and extended versions, which are produced by varying the width of the letters. Each variation affects legibility.

THIS IS LIGHT.

THIS IS MEDIUM.

THIS IS BOLD.

THIS IS CONDENSED.

THIS IS STANDARD (ROMAN).

THIS IS EXTENDED.

Letter Size

For outdoor signs on highways and city streets, it is recommended that lettering be no less than 4 inches (10 centimeters) high where vehicle speeds are 30 to 35 miles per hour (50 to 55 kilometers per hour). For speeds over 40 miles per hour (65 kilometers per hour), 5-inch (12.5-centimeter) lettering is preferable.

The accompanying table will serve as an aid in determining the correct letter size for sign legibility for both internally illuminated signs and opaque signs that will be illuminated by spotlights or ambient light. Other factors, such as obstructions to view, the distance from which the sign will be read, whether it will be read from a moving vehicle and at what speed, and the number of signs in a particular location, must be taken into account; thus, judgment of the particular situation is important.

In addition to letter size, other factors that contribute to sign legibility include the number of characters per line, the number of words per sign, and the percentage of the face of the sign occupied by lettering. As a general rule, the length of a line should not exceed one alphabet (26 characters, including spaces); no more than 16 words should appear on a sign; no more than 50 percent of any sign face should be occupied by verbal messages, including words and numbers.

Certain messages require more emphasis than others. This can be achieved by several means: using larger letters; using all capital letters; changing weight or color; or changing type style, for example, from roman to italic letters.

RELATIONSHIP OF LETTER HEIGHT TO VIEWING DISTANCE FOR OPAQUE AND INTERNALLY LIGHTED SIGNS

Letter Height		Viewing Distance			
		Opaque Letters		Internally Lighted Letters	
Inches	Centi-meters	Feet	Meters	Feet	Meters
24	60	840	256	1,200	366
12	30	420	128	600	183
6	15	210	64	300	91
2	5	70	21	100	30
1	2.5	35	11	40	12

Layout

Sign design is usually considered in terms of modules. Modules of various sizes can be combined to convey a variety of information, such as floor number, room number, occupant's name, direction, and so forth. The size of the module should be determined by the frequency of use and the greatest distance from which it must be legible. Attractive design can be an element in choosing layout, as long as legibility is paramount.

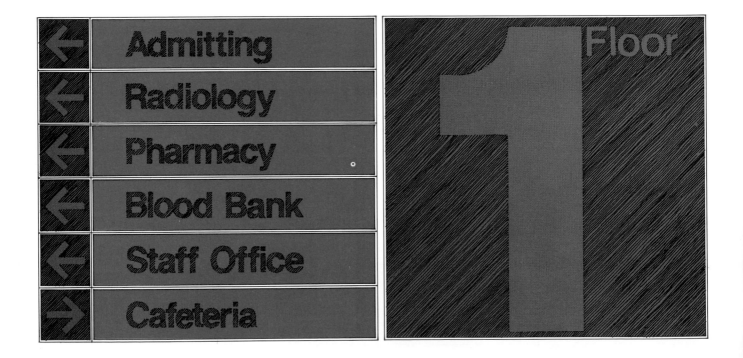

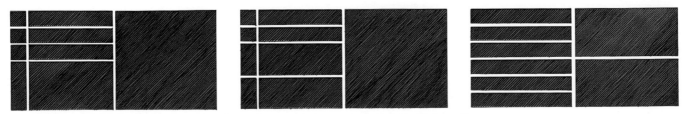

Modules of various sizes can be combined into sign panels to convey a variety of information.

Individual modules lend flexibility to a sign system, because they can be rearranged or changed easily. Under some circumstances, it is desirable to combine individual modules to produce wall layouts or freestanding signs. For example, multiple assemblies can be constructed by using single modules in quantity. Emphasis can be achieved through a creative arrangement of modules, and blank modules can act as linear spaces for greater legibility.

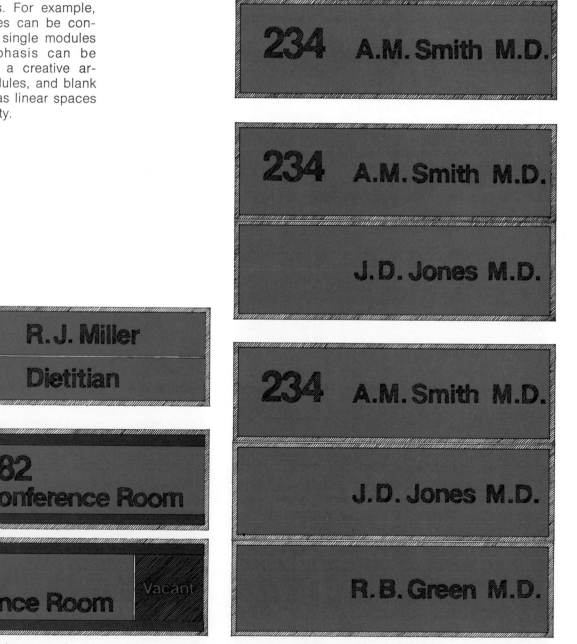

Individual modules can be arranged or changed as needed. Signs that can be shifted to indicate when rooms are in use provide additional flexibility.

Another way to achieve emphasis is to use different type sizes, according to the legibility requirements and the function of the message.

The length of the message to be conveyed often determines the size of the type and of the sign. Crucial messages should be short, one word, if possible, in order to give them the most emphasis. It is better to put the single word "Emergency" in large letters on a sign than "Emergency Entrance" or, worse, "Turn Right for Emergency Entrance." Similarly, the word "Stop" can be emphasized more easily than "Please Stop at Gate" and much more easily than "Please Stop at Gate Before Proceeding to Admitting Desk."

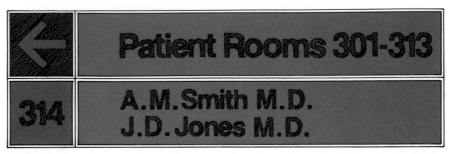

Different type sizes can be used on one size of panel, according to the legibility requirements and the function of the message.

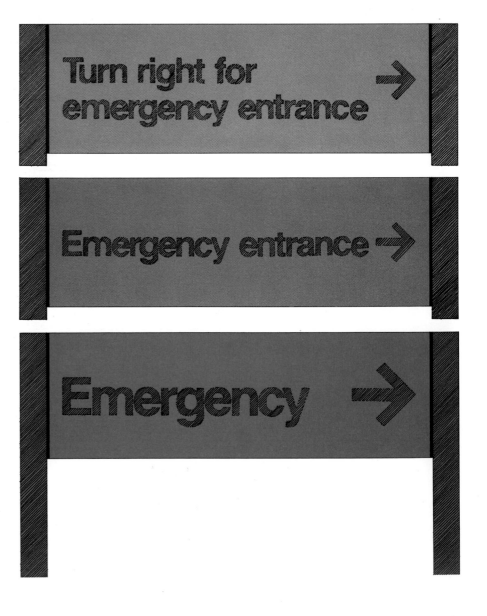

Crucial messages should consist of one word, if possible, in order to give them emphasis.

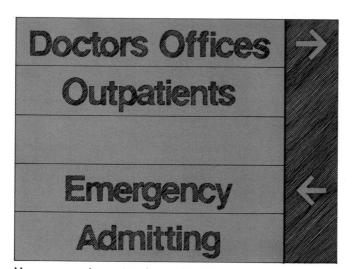

Messages can be centered on a sign panel.

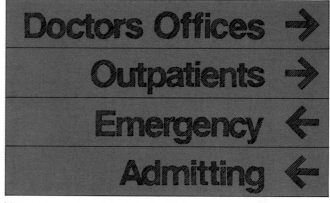

Messages can be aligned flush right.

When a number of messages must be included on the same sign panel, several choices of layout are possible. If several words or phrases are to be combined on a sign panel, they can be centered, aligned with a left-hand margin (called flush left), or aligned with a right-hand margin (called flush right). The flush-left arrangement is the most common and the most easily read in Western cultures. Flush-left and flush-right arrangements of words appear more orderly and therefore more legible than a centered arrangement and are preferred.

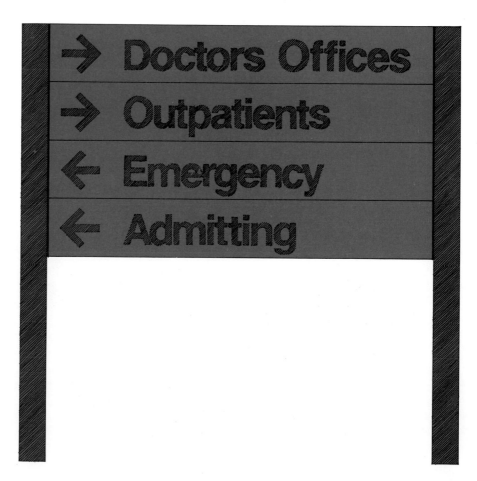

Flush-left arrangement of messages is preferred.

Placement

Signs can be affixed to the plane of the walls, using a number of types of brackets or other fasteners; they can be attached to wall brackets so as to project at right angles from the wall; they can be mounted on standards or easels vertical to the floor; or they can be hung from the ceiling. Any combination of mountings can be used throughout the system. Choices will depend upon such factors as architecture, ceiling height, visibility, major traffic flow, and so forth. If large signs, in particular, are to be hung from the structural ceiling, the placement of pipes, beams, or other obstructions that may be above a false ceiling and that could interfere with sign placement must be considered.

The height at which a sign is placed is critical. In general, for interior signs on the plane of the wall the area from 5 to 7 feet above the floor is a convenient "information zone" for most users. For maximum legibility signs need as much open space surrounding them as does the lettering on the sign panel; that is, no more than 50 percent of the wall space in the information zone should be occupied by signs. Mounting signs at a uniform height, even though ceiling heights may differ from one location to another, helps to create a cohesive appearance.

For signs that project from the plane of the wall or are hung from the ceiling, the bottom edge of the sign should be at least 7 feet above the floor to allow headroom and room for the movement of equipment such as intravenous fluid stands. Care should be taken that brackets and signs do not obscure nurse call lights over patient room doors.

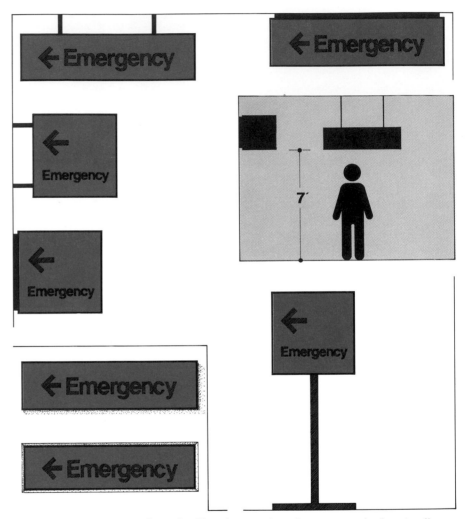

Signs can be affixed to walls and ceilings in a number of ways or can be freestanding. When signs are suspended from a ceiling or project from a wall, there should be a minimum clearance of 7 feet above the floor.

7

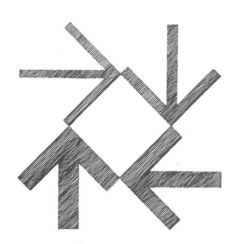

ACQUIRING SIGNS

All efforts to this point have been preliminary. The next step is to choose the elements of the sign system; typefaces, sizes, colors, and methods of installation. In short, all the final decisions must now be made. These decisions will be made together with the consultant, if one has been retained. Consultants often have a "preferred list" of qualified manufacturers and should assist the hospital in the selection of appropriate manufacturers to bid on projects. If there is no consultant, sign manufacturers must be contacted direct.

The best source of preliminary information about major sign manufacturers is *Sweet's Architectural Catalog File.** Also useful are the classified pages of the telephone directory; sign manufacturers who not only do custom work but also act as area representatives for major sign manufacturing companies are located in all large cities and most small cities and towns.

It is essential to carefully check the qualifications of consultants and manufacturers, and the following recommendations apply to both. Time spent now can save time, money, and irritation later.† If at all possible, hospital representatives should visit other institutions that have completed and installed sign projects done by the consultants or manufacturers who are under consideration. The rep-

---

*Available in business departments of public libraries.

†Interviews of graphic consultants and sign manufacturers can be conducted on much the same basis as those of architects. See *Selection of Architects for Health Facility Projects,* published by the American Hospital Association, Chicago, 1975.

resentatives should ask questions: On what basis did the client work with the consultant? Did the manufacturer or supplier meet the required time schedule? Was the cost of installation for all the signs, or for only some of them, included in the bid price? Was the work satisfactory?

The quality of the signs themselves should be studied: Are the letters clean-cut? Are all elements smooth-edged? How well was the installation done? Are the colors uniform?

Also, the integrity of the system should be studied: Is it consistent throughout? Can it be changed easily?

If personal visits to completed projects are not possible, the consultant or manufacturer should be asked for references among his clients, and these clients should be contacted.

Three or four of the manufacturers under consideration can be asked to supply actual prototypes of the kinds of signs that might be ordered. These can be used in lieu of the homemade mock-ups, mentioned in chapter 5, for testing appearance and legibility under actual conditions of use.

Costs and Budgeting

What with variations in type, quality, size, location, and other factors, reliable budget figures for a hospital sign system are virtually impossible to tie down. There is no formula for computing the cost—no cost-per-bed or cost-per-square-foot figure. The materials specified and the fabrication techniques required are the major cost determinants. Engraving on plastic laminate is the least expensive; fiber-reinforced plastic the most costly. Hot-stamping or silk-screening on plastic or aluminum panels is in the middle price range. Signs with subsurface printing are least likely to be vandalized, and for some institutions this could justify some additional original cost.

The use of stock signs wherever possible and of stock sizes for the materials selected can also lower the cost. Sheets of clear, rigid plastic are produced in standard sizes up to 6 feet by 8 feet; if signs are cut in even multiples rather than in odd sizes, savings in the cost of materials will result, as there will be little waste or spoilage of material.

As businesses and institutions have become more aware of the advantages of good informational sign systems, more consultants and manufacturers have entered the field. Because of this increased competition, owners should shop carefully among suppliers to be sure of the best value. If the work of charting the messages, placement, and quantities of signs needed has been done thoroughly, the fabricator will be able to give an estimate of the cost of deluxe, medium-range, or budget jobs and of the kind of system the hospital can expect in each price range. If the sign system will be the major interior design element and the primary means of introducing visual interest, the additional cost of the highest-quality signs is justified.

If the services of a designer or graphic consultant are used, his fee must be considered. This may be a separate consulting fee, or, if the designer is retained to carry through the total system, the price will include his professional fee and the cost of fabrication and installation.

If signs are to be ordered and installed in phases or their manufacture held in abeyance, the bid figures may not continue to be valid.

Funds for developing and implementing a sign system should not come out of operating budgets, but should be treated as a capital expenditure, just like renovation or new construction. If this is not done, it will be difficult to enlist the cooperation of all departments from whose budgets the money must come. Although it is easier to include a sign system in the capital budget when a hospital is being built or when a major expansion is under way, it is just as essential to do so whether or not the hospital is in a building program.

The designer or sign fabricator should be asked to furnish a payment schedule stipulating when deposits and final payments are due. This is necessary for cash-flow projections.

Taking Bids and Ordering

To make sure of getting the signs that have been decided on, a detailed specification document that leaves no room for speculation or substitutions—that is, no "or equal" clauses—should be prepared. The specification document is assurance of getting what you want.

The Construction Specifications Institute* has developed an outline of specifications pertaining to signs.

"Drawings

"Show site plan locations of signs, elevations, dimensions, height above ground, construction details; layout of design to include letter heights, composition and spacing of listings, logotypes, size of perspective if used; and, should illumination be required, the location and number of lights, the source of power, and controls.

"Specifications

"Cover the installation and maintenance of signs, quality of materials, qualifications of sign painter, the number of colors required, listings of titles, names, if illumination is required, the hours of operation and responsibility for payment of power used; and the complete removal of [temporary] signs at the completion of the project."

*Construction Specifications Institute, 1150 17th St., N.W., Washington, DC 20036.

If a consultant prepares the specification document, it becomes the property of the institution once it is complete. Five to 10 copies will be needed, depending on the size of the project. If the sign program is undertaken as part of a construction project, the general contractor will need copies. One copy will be needed for each vendor bidding, and there should be at least two copies each for the administration and for the hospital's purchasing department. Copies of the final specification document should be retained by the hospital for use in ordering new or replacement signs.

For an existing facility, ordering and taking of bids should be handled through the purchasing department. If the facility is new, the architect, consultant, or construction manager can do this. In some cases ordering and bidding are specified in the architect's contract and will be charged for as part of his services. For projects of more than $100,000, bid bonds and financial statements should be required.

Invitations to bid must be sent to all bidders at the same time. It is recommended that at least three but not more than five vendors be invited to bid. Three satisfies government bidding procedures; more than five can discourage interest and, therefore, thoughtful and competitive bids. A specific date and time for bid opening must also be announced; keep in mind that manufacturers need two to three weeks to prepare bids.

Invitations to bid should also stipulate exactly how price information is to be stated. This is particularly important if the budget is tight and cutbacks might be necessary. Pricing breakdowns can be by sign categories, areas, and/or floor levels.

The invitation to bid should state whether the bid is for fabrication only and/or for installation of all or some of the signs. Installation by the manufacturer, if the budget permits and if he has the capability, can eliminate headaches about shipment of signs to the site and the handling and care of the signs before they are installed.

Installation of signs can be quite costly. A rule of thumb puts the cost at 15 to 20 percent of total sign cost. An extensive exterior system, with many internally illuminated or spotlighted signs, may require conduit or complex electrical installations beyond the capability of the hospital's own building and grounds department. Large freestanding outdoor signs usually require embedding in cement blocks two or three feet below grade, which may call for heavy digging and leveling equipment. Generally, such signs should not be installed in cold regions during the winter when the work is more difficult and more expensive. Such installation should be guided by local conditions and ordinances.

Installation of most interior signs can be handled by a good maintenance department. Wall-mounted signs at eye level should present few problems. Whether the signs are bolted to the wall or affixed by chemical adhesives, not much is needed beyond a ruler, a level, and an accurate eye. Ceiling-mounted signs, however, can present more complex installation problems because of the need to avoid piping and ductwork.

If installation is not included in the manufacturer's bid and is not within the capability of the hospital's own personnel, a separate contract with a local installer will be required. Sign manufacturers should provide drawings and installation instructions for all types of signs in order to allow the client to decide whether in-house installation is feasible.

If a consultant is used, the consultant should read the bids and advise the client on which is the best choice. The lowest bid should not automatically get the job. Past performance (judged on personal observations or recommendations of previous clients, or both), current work load, and ability to meet the schedule should all be considered in addition to price.

Delivery

A specific date for delivery, or completion of installation, if that is included, should be made part of the contract, together with an agreed-upon penalty amount for every day the delivery or installation schedule slips. Eight to 10 weeks should be allowed for fabrication of interior signs, and 12 to 15 weeks for exterior signs. The manufacturer should notify the client well in advance if he foresees any problem in meeting the specified delivery date.

Shipping can take as long as two or three weeks, depending on the distance and the method of shipment. Provisions should be made ahead of time for receiving, uncrating, and checking the signs for accuracy in meeting specifications and for damage. The hospital is responsible for checking the condition of the signs and for filing damage claims. If the hospital does not have adequate storage space, arrangements may have to be made with a local company to store large exterior signs.

If a consultant has been retained, he should have provided a location drawing for all signs and should be at the site during installation, if at all possible, to make sure that the signs are accurate and that they are installed at the right location. A final check of the fabrication and the installation should be completed by the consultant and a hospital representative together.

In-House Systems

The possibility of fabricating some signs in-house was mentioned briefly in chapter 6. Sometimes it is preferable for a hospital to use a total in-house system. For example, an urban hospital with several buildings on a tight site, where departments are constantly being shifted and the use of space is often changed, might find this to be the only practical approach.

Information gathering, design criteria, placement of the signs, and the other procedures and considerations mentioned earlier apply equally in the case of a system that is to be fabricated in-house.

Because the sign-making process will be a continuing one, a special area should be set aside for it, preferably near the printing and carpentry shops. The space should be adequate for one or two persons and for all equipment, supplies, and inventory of signs on hand. Equipment and materials that are used frequently in sign fabrication include an engraving machine, vinyl letters, sheets of clear rigid plastic, fiberboard, and printing equipment.

If the system is to be fabricated in-house, it is imperative that it be well thought out and well designed, and thoroughly documented in a manual of procedures. Many graphics consultants are prepared to design systems that can be handled in this way.

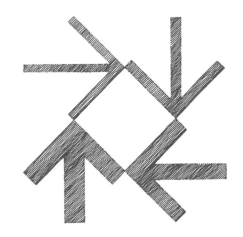

NUMBERING SYSTEMS

Basically, there are two types of numbering systems in every institution. One is used to direct patient, staff, and visitor traffic; the other is used only by staff and maintenance personnel for keeping track of furniture and equipment inventories, painting schedules, and location of electrical facilities, telephone closets, and other utility areas.

This does not mean that every space must have a number on or beside its door. Such spaces as janitors' closets and electrical and telephone closets should be identified on the plans maintained by the building engineer, so that maintenance personnel and electrical or telephone repair personnel can locate these areas from the plans. However, many institutions find it simpler to physically mark each space. This can be done with small unobtrusive numbers for all spaces that do not need to be identified for the public.

Architectural drawings generally have every space numbered in order to identify spaces relative to finish, equipment, door, and other schedules. It is helpful if the initial numbering system and the ultimate room numbering system are the same or are coordinated. In an existing building, the numbering on the plans may not conform to the room numbering system, and in such cases the plans should be renumbered.

A numbering system should be as easy as possible to understand by persons who are unfamiliar with the facility. Whether in inpatient care areas or in outpatient and ambulatory care areas, numbering systems should always be started as close as possible to the entry point—the lobby, the outpatient entrance, or the elevators. A room numbering system should never be started from a point that has no direct reference to where people enter the hospital or the area.

It is strongly suggested that no more than four digits be used in a room numbering system; three digits are preferable. This is particularly important if patient-room telephones are to be coordinated with room numbers, because most telephone systems will not accommodate more than three digits for extensions.

All spaces that require public access ought to carry numbers or other identification on or next to their corridor doors. In nursing units, patient-room numbers should be visible when the door is open; therefore it is preferable to place them on the wall next to the door and on the side opposite the door hinge. Other rooms, such as toilet rooms or staff work areas where doors are normally kept closed, can carry an identification on the door itself.

The most common practice is to number rooms by levels. Floor level designation should start at the entrance level, and numbers above and below should support the main level designation. Thus, all numbers on the first level can begin with the digit 1, on the second level with 2, and so on. Rooms on floors below the first (or lobby) level can use such prefixes as B (basement), G (ground), SB (subbasement), or 01, 02, and so on. If parking is located on these levels, the prefixes P1, P2, and so forth are often used.

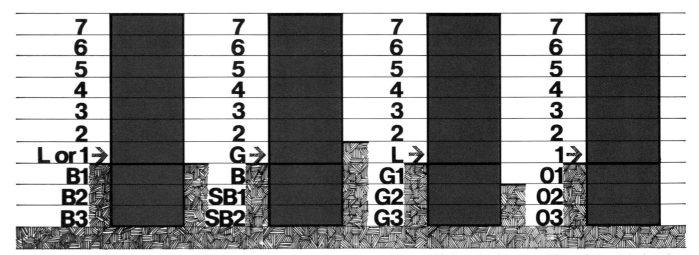

The designation of floor level should start at the entrance level; numbers above and below should support the main level designation.

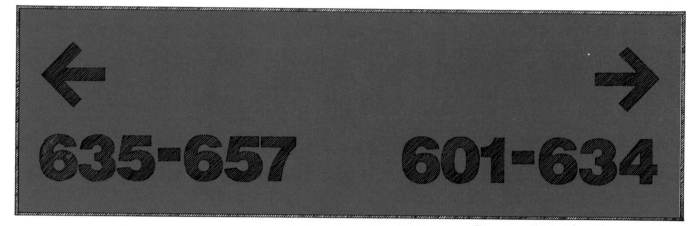

Room numbering in patient care areas can be simplified if the numbers constitute a series starting from each side of each traffic concentration point.

Finding the location of a particular room in patient care areas can be simplified if the numbers constitute a continuous series on each side of each traffic entry point.

The simplest numbering system along a corridor is serial, with even numbers on the right and odd numbers on the left. If a short subcorridor angles off from the main corridor, the numbering can continue along the subcorridor, continuing the odd or even numbers for that particular side of the main corridor. Thus, a small sign at the cross corridor can indicate that rooms 612 and 614 open off the subcorridor.

Considerable discretion must be used for room numbering. For example, the simple system already described may not be adaptable to a situation where a long subcorridor exists on only one side of the main corridor, because the odd-numbered and even-numbered sides would be out of balance with each other.

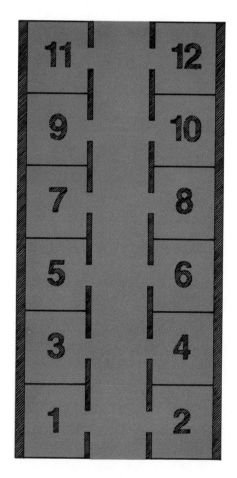

The simplest numbering system along a corridor is consecutive, with even numbers on the right and odd numbers on the left in relation to the starting point.

When rooms are situated around a central core, they also can be numbered consecutively. The rooms may form a U shape, a circle, or a rectangle, and if there are rooms within the core, these can be included in the numbering system.

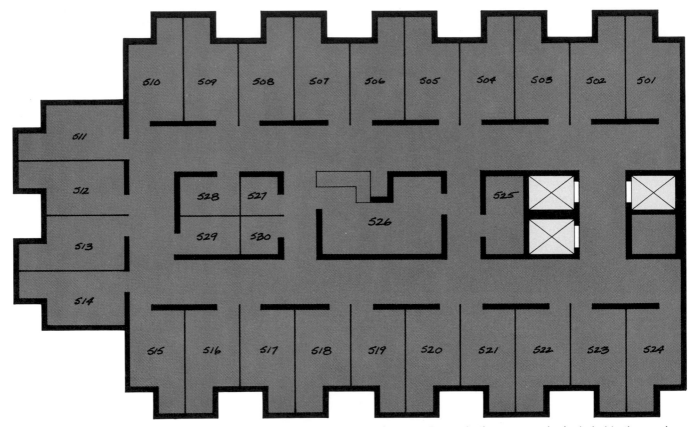

Rooms in a U-shaped corridor can be numbered consecutively around the core. Rooms in the core can be included in the numbering system.

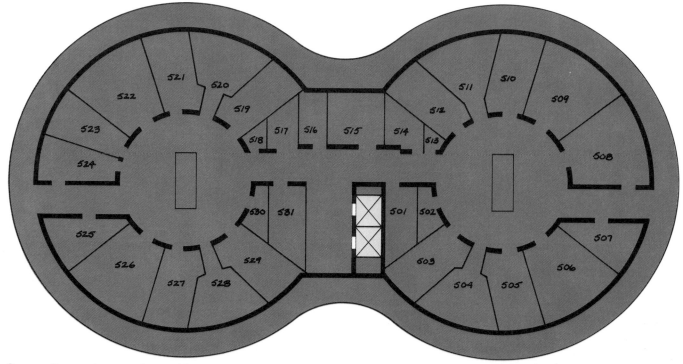

Consecutive numbers can be used for rooms on twin floor layouts.

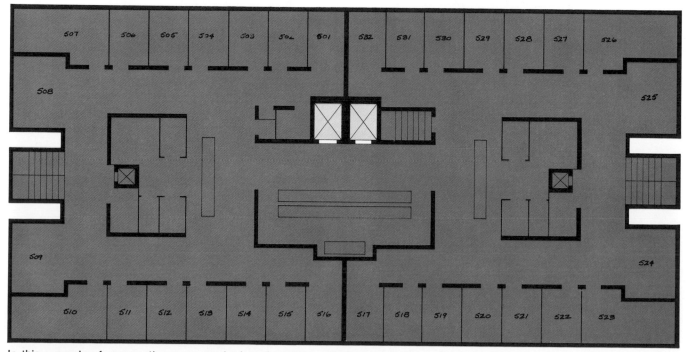

In this example of consecutive room numbering, the traffic entry point is at the center of the floor.

Another room numbering system consists of designating patient rooms by one series of numbers, either odd or even. All rooms used by the staff and service personnel should then be numbered by the alternate series.

In a complex layout, or in a facility with several wings or buildings, a letter prefix to the number may be necessary, such as W101 for room 101 in the West Wing, or E101 for room 101 in the East Wing. Color coding can be useful in this situation, as noted earlier.

If a room has more than one door opening off the corridor, all doors should be given the same number. For numbering rooms within rooms, a letter suffix is generally used, for example, 109a, 109b, and so forth. Toilet rooms or bathrooms within patient rooms do not require numbers. Large conference and demonstration rooms that can be divided by folding partitions and that have several doors can be identified as, for instance, 110A (conference) and 110B (demonstration).

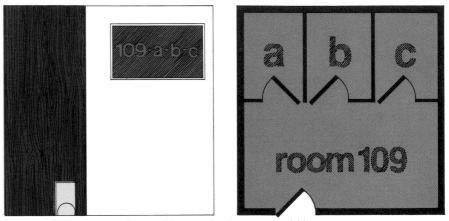

A letter suffix is generally used for numbering rooms within rooms.

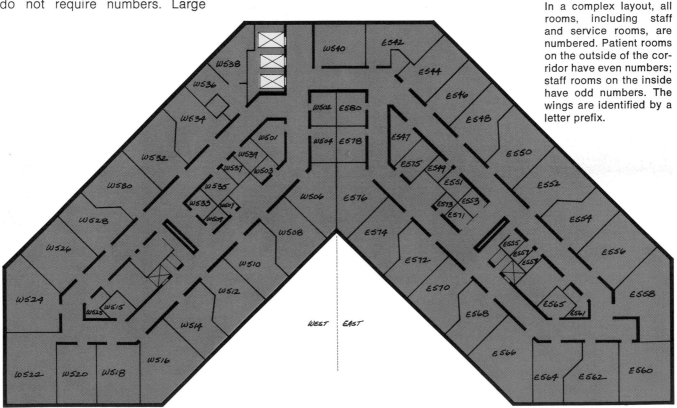

In a complex layout, all rooms, including staff and service rooms, are numbered. Patient rooms on the outside of the corridor have even numbers; staff rooms on the inside have odd numbers. The wings are identified by a letter prefix.

9

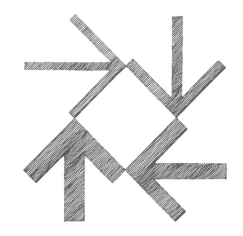

MAINTAINING THE SYSTEM

The signs have been constructed and installed. The job is over. Well, not quite. Time, effort, and money have been invested in developing the signs and graphics system. Now, like any other part of the hospital's buildings and equipment, the system has to be maintained.

Overall responsibility for maintenance should be given to one person. This may be someone in the administrator's office or in the engineering or purchasing departments. At this stage, the design consultant should turn over to the person designated the manual of technical data concerning the system. This information will be needed to order new or replacement signs. It is most important that sizes, forms, and colors be consistent with the original system, so that it is maintained as it was first conceived.

Temporary Signs

Temporary signs may be required while replacements for permanent signs are on order. They may also be needed until permanent signs are installed upon the completion of each construction phase where the signs program has been phased in over a period, or during a period when the hospital is undergoing renovation or piecemeal expansion. Because construction often creates the need for temporary entrances, exits, and routing patterns, the need for signs is usually acute. If temporary signs are used in conjunction with a permanent sign system, the style of the temporary signs should conform as closely as possible to the permanent ones.

For temporary exterior signs, the least expensive method is generally to have them painted by a local sign painter. Attention must always be paid to the design, the color, and the style of letters used. Such signs can be spotlighted at night.

For the interior, painted fiberboard is one inexpensive solution. Or the hospital may consider buying an inexpensive engraving machine. Although not totally satisfactory from an esthetic standpoint, such a device can be valuable in the in-house fabrication of a low-cost temporary system. Paper signs, either in neat hand lettering or carefully applied rub-on letters, sandwiched between clear plastic panels, can also be used as a temporary expedient. These materials are available in a number of sizes off the shelf in art supply stores. Vinyl letters, available in a variety of alphabets, sizes, and colors, can be lined up with the help of a spacing guide to form messages. Such letters make attractive temporary signs, but they are not cheap and they are not vandal-proof—a fact that should be considered in terms of their placement and the incidence of vandalism at the particular institution. Temporary signs can be suspended from ceilings on thin wires so as not to damage wall surfaces.

Maintenance Procedures

Written procedures should be developed for sign maintenance, as for any other function. The person responsible should schedule a complete tour of the facility every three or four months. Such a tour should be made with a critical eye for deficiencies, which can include such items as damaged signs, signs that have come loose from walls or standards, and signs that are out of date with regard to the areas or personnel they designate.

The person in charge of maintaining the system should also be alert to trouble spots. Just because a sign has been installed does not mean that it is doing its job. He should also watch for "additions" to the sign system in the form of signs put up by staff members. Such visual static not only can ruin the most well-thought-out system, but also can be an indication of a trouble spot.

When room assignments are changed, new personnel are hired, or areas are remodeled, the person responsible for sign maintenance should ensure that all necessary new signs are ordered and installed and should notify all departments of the changes.

Special forms can be used by department heads for requesting new signs, but no one except the individual designated should place the order. This is imperative if the new signs are to be ordered in the appropriate typefaces, sizes, and colors in order to preserve the integrity of the system.

The person responsible for sign maintenance should discuss the handling of new and replacement orders with the sign fabricator. It is helpful if the fabricator keeps a file on the project at his office, and it is important for the responsible staff person to know what information the fabricator will need to process reorders, how long replacement will take, and to what extent costs can be expected to remain stable in the future.

Most important, the commitment of the administrator to the signs and graphics project must be carried through to the maintenance phase, or much of the early work will have gone for naught. The system will be only as good as the maintenance process is thorough.

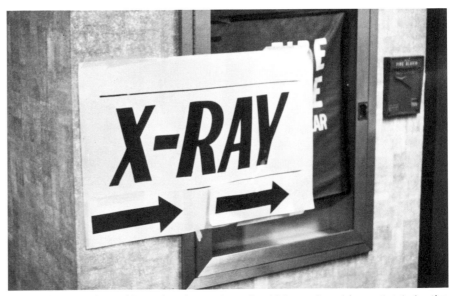

An addition such as this to the sign system should be replaced immediately by the maintenance department.

BIBLIOGRAPHY

American Hospital Association. *Uniform Hospital Definitions.* Chicago: AHA, 1960.

American Institute of Architects. *Accessibility—The Law and Reality. A Survey to Test the Application and Effectiveness of Public Law 90-480 in Iowa.* Des Moines, IA: AIA Iowa Chapter, 1974.

American Institute of Graphic Arts. *Symbol Signs* (Publication DOT-05040192). Prepared for the Office of Facilitation, U.S. Dept. of Transportation. National Technical Information Service, Springfield, VA 22151.

American National Standards Institute. *ANSI Standard D6.-1971. Manual on Uniform Traffic Control Devices.* New York City: ANSI, 1971.

_____. *ANSI Standard Z35.1-1972. Specifications for Accident Prevention Signs.* New York City: ANSI, 1972.

Arnell, A. *Standard Graphical Symbols: A Comprehensive Guide for Use in Industry, Engineering, and Science.* New York City: McGraw-Hill Book Co., 1963.

Arthur P. Sunnybrook Hospital's new information system. *Canadian Hospital.* 45:41, Feb. 1968.

Bright, bold sign program directs people through hospital: Massachusetts Eye and Ear Infirmary. *Hospitals, J.A.H.A.* 49:25, Feb. 1, 1975.

Cahn, J. G. Graphic Rx for a hospital: is half a dose better than none? *Print.* 25:56, Mar.-Apr. 1971.

Camp, G. van, and Rensbergen, van. Visuele signalisatie en geschreven communicatie in ziekenhuizen. [Signposting and written communications in the hospital.] *Acta Hospitalia* (Louvain). 10:36, 1970. Summary in French.

Clipson, C. W. Public information systems giving the patient the information he needs. *Hosp. Bldg. and Eng.* (London). 3:17, May 1970.

Crosby/Fletcher/Forbes. *A Sign Systems Manual.* New York City: Praeger, 1970.

De Goey, J. Effective graphics system: more than meets the eye. *Building Oper. Manage.* 21:20, July 1974.

De Neve, R. Signs and symbols for a children's hospital. *Print.* 26:26, Mar. 1972.

Dornette, W. H. L., and Bartlett, L. A. System identifies fire-hazard areas. *Hosp. Top.* 48:31, July 1970.

Dreyfuss, H. *Symbol Sourcebook: An Authoritative Guide to International Graphic Symbols.* New York City: McGraw-Hill Book Co., 1972.

Eisenberg, A. M., and Smith, R. R. *Nonverbal Communications* (Speech Communication Series, no. 9). New York City: Bobbs, 1972.

Expandable hospital stretches to fit medical needs of area's population. *Mod. Hosp.* 118:88, Feb. 1972.

Freeway motorists now will see hospital signs. *Mich. Med.* 71:600, July 1972.

Graphics ease eye patients through hospital. *Hospitals, J.A.H.A.* 50:35, May 16, 1976.

Harney, A. L. Signage: fitting letter forms to building form. *Amer. Inst. Architects J.* 64:35, Oct. 1975.

Highway signs to identify emergency medical services facilities urged. *AID.* 6:6, Oct. 1971.

Hoffman, P. Signs tell patients where to go. *Mod. Healthcare.* 5:51, Mar. 1976.

Hospital directional signs under study. *Hosp. Forum* (NY). 38:2, Dec. 1970.

Hospital graphics. *Ind. Des.* 19:58, Apr. 1972.

Klumb (E. Christopher) Associates. *Architectural Graphics Manual: Signage Standards for Health Facilities of the City of New York.* New York City: E. Christopher Klumb Associates, 1971.

Klumb, E. C. Hospital signs that everyone can understand. *Mod. Hosp.* 120:96, May 1973.

Knight, R. S., and Bartels, D. H. Effective signage: systems approach to smooth traffic flow. *Building Oper. Manage.* 22:18, Sept. 1975.

Lipper, C. Good signs can help control visitor and staff traffic. *Mod. Hosp.* 115:83, July 1970.

Not that way (Film). Chicago: American Hospital Association, 1975.

Occupational Safety and Health Administration. *General Industry Standards and Interpretations.* Washington, DC: Superintendent of Documents, U.S. Government Printing Office. Available by subscription or from OSHA regional offices.

Olson, D. R. What we need is another sign. *Med. Group. Manage.* 20:18, Mar.-Apr. 1973.

Osman, M. E. Substitutes for words. *Amer. Hist. Architect. J.* 58:3, Aug. 1972.

Owens, J. Travelers need signs locating hospital care. *Mod. Hosp.* 106:95, Apr. 1966.

Page, M. Signs and symbols for health facilities. *Interiors.* 131:16, Feb. 1972.

Pictographs to guide hospital visitors. *Hospitals, J.A.H.A.* 46:109, Jan. 1, 1972.

Planning, flexibility, and growth enable hospitals' signage systems to meet many needs. *Hospitals, J.A.H.A.* 51:54, July 16, 1977.

Pollet. D. L. New Directions in library signage. *Wilson Lib. Bull.* 50:456, Feb. 1976.

Pollet, D. L., and Haskell, P. H., editors. *Wayfinding: Designing Sign Systems for Libraries.* New York City: R. R. Bowker Co. Summer 1979.

Ruiz, G. G. Information systems for The Child Hospital of Buenos Aires. *Novum Gebrauchsgraphik.* 46:44, Jan. 1975.

Signage system eases frustration: Mount Sinai Medical Center, Chicago. *Hospitals, J.A.H.A.* 48:50, Apr. 16, 1974.

Signs guide motorists to Illinois trauma centers. *Hospitals, J.A.H.A.* 46:121, Aug. 16, 1972.

Smith, C. N. Sign systems, with special emphasis on use in medical facilities. *Int. Des.* 46:148, Oct. 1975.

Smith, S. B. Graphics in Maine hospitals. *J. Maine Med. Assn.* 65:63, Mar. 1974.

Steinle, J. G. Many mechanical and visual methods of visitor control are used in hospitals. *Hosp. Top.* 53:11, Mar.-Apr. 1976.

Torpy, T. F. Graphic symbols in an occupational health service. *J. Occup. Med.* 17:756, Dec. 1975.

Traffic in hospitals. *Architect. and Eng. News.* 9:74, July 1967.

U.S. Department of Housing and Urban Development. *The Urban Signage Forum, April 22 and 23, 1976, Chicago, Illinois. Proceedings.* Washington, DC: Superintendent of Documents, U.S. Government Printing office.

Veterans Administration, Office of Construction. *Directional Graphics for VA Hospitals.* Washington, DC: Superintendent of Documents, U.S. Government Printing Office, 1976. Price $2.10.

Visual communications. *Ind. Des.* 22:64, May 1975.

Visual signs at Memorial Hospital of Long Beach, Calif. *Hosp. Top.* 48:20, Oct. 1970.

Voort, A. P. F. van der. Bewegwitzering in en om gebouwen. [Signposting in and around buildings.] *Instelling-Management (Den Haag).* 5:193, Apr. 1973.

Webster, L. F. Super graphics point the way at Etobicoke General Hospital. *Hosp. Admin. Can.* 15:58, May 1973.

Which way? Architectural graphics should direct or inform the user. *Architect. and Eng. News.* 11:21, Mar. 1969.

Which way to purchasing? Hospitals are experimenting with new signs. *Amer. Surg. Dealer.* 60:88, Sept. 1973.

Wittrup, R. How to number hospital rooms. *Hospitals, J.A.H.A.* 32:53, Sept. 1, 1958.

INDEX

Access roads, in site planning, 14
Acquiring signs
  checking quality, 52
  checking suppliers, 51-52
  from manufacturers, 51-54
Advisory signs, illus., 36
Alarming signs, placement, 19
Approaches, planning and identifying, 7-11
Approaches to site, planning for, 7
Approach road, planning, 9, illus., 9
Architect, role, 4
Atrium, in orienting building users, 19
Audible/tactile signs, for visually
  handicapped, 11

■ ■ ■

Building, as communicator, 4
Building design, coordinated with signs
  and graphics, 5
Building numbering, checklist, 34
Building planning, related to movement
  of traffic, 5
Building user groups. See User groups
Bus stops, need for signs, illus., 11
Bus and subway stops. See Public
  transportation stops

■ ■ ■

Cautionary signs, illus., 36
Checklist for interior planning, 20-21
Checklist for site planning, 14-15
Color, use in signs, 40
Community, served by signs and graphics
  system, 4
Construction Specifications
  Institute, 53
Coordinator, of sign committee, 23
Corridors
  directional signs, 32, illus., 32, 33
  room numbering systems, 57, illus.,
  57, 58
Corridor schemes, planning for, 19
Cultural differences, in understanding
  symbols and pictographs, 38

■ ■ ■

Data collection
  checklist, 34
  cooperation of staff members, 26
  plotting the information, 26-31
  for signs and graphics system, 23,
  25-26
  statement of existing conditions, 26
Delivery and service personnel, served
  by signs and graphics system, 3
Design of signs, 46-49, illus., 46, 47,
  48, 49

Desirable traffic patterns, communication
  of, 5
Directional signs
  on approach walks, 13
  at entrances, 13
  near public transportation stops, 11
Doors
  identification, 32
  signs and identification, 19

■ ■ ■

Elevator, in multistoried parking
  structure, 13
Emergency department
  interior planning, 21
  reception and waiting areas, 19
  secondary drives, 9
  served by signs and graphics
  system, 4
Emergency department entrance
  preceding main entrance drive, 7-8
  reception control point for, 10
  in site planning, 15
Emergency drives, design, 10
Emergency entrance, design features,
  illus., 10
Employee parking, location, 12
Entrance drive, signs for, 7, 8
Entrances, in site planning, 15
Existing health care facility, need
  for signs and graphics
  system, 4
Existing signs, in new system, 4
Exterior signs, checklist, 34

■ ■ ■

Grouping departments in interior
  planning, 17-18, illus., 18

■ ■ ■

Handicapped persons
  ramps, 12
  in site planning, 14
  special sign requirements, 25
Health care facility, master plan for
  signs and graphics, 4
Highway signs, U.S. Department of
  Transportation, 39
Hospital building complex, visual
  identification, 6
Hospital building plans
  related to user groups, 26-28, illus., 28
  simplified drawings, 26-29, illus., 27
Hospital departments, in plans and
  drawings, 26-29
Hospital floor levels, room numbering
  systems, 55-56, illus., 56
Hospital identity, signs for, 7

Hospital staff, served by signs and
  graphics system, 3, 4
Hospital user groups. See User groups

■ ■ ■

Identification signs, illus., 36
Identifying signs
  on approach walks, 13
  at entrances, 13
Information signs, illus., 36
Information system
  choosing messages, 35-40
  media, 35-40
  symbols and pictographs, 37-40,
  illus., 37, 38
  terminology, 35-36
Interior planning
  checklist, 20-21
  design principles, 17-19
  desirable traffic patterns, 28-30
  emergency department, 20
  functional areas, 21
  grouping departments, 17-18, illus., 18
  main entrance lobby, 20
  outpatient department, 20
  patient floors, 21
  traffic movement, 17-19
Interior signs, checklist, 34

■ ■ ■

Layout of signs, 46-49, illus., 46, 47,
  48, 49

■ ■ ■

Main entrance
  approach to, 7
  identification, 10, illus., 10
  secondary drives, 9
  in site planning, 15
Main entrance drive
  planning, 7-8
  separated from parking areas, 12
  signs for, 8
Main entrance lobby, interior planning, 20
Maintenance, of signs, 61-62
Marking, for areas and facilities,
  planning checklist, 20-21
Media, in information system, 35-40
Medical staff, served by signs and
  graphics system, 3
Movement signs, illus., 36
Multistoried parking structure. See
  Parking structure

■ ■ ■

National Fire Protection Association,
  special symbols, 39
New health care facility, need for signs
  and graphics system 4

"No Parking" signs, at entrances, 13
"No Smoking" signs
    placement, 19
    pictograph for, 38, illus., 38
Numbering systems, for rooms, 55-60,
        illus., 56, 57, 58, 59, 60
Nursing staff, served by signs and
        graphics system, 3

■ ■ ■

OSHA. See Occupational Safety and
        Health Administration
Occupational Safety and Health
        Administration
    requirements, 25
    use of color in signs, 40
Onsite pedestrian traffic, in site
        planning, 15
Onsite traffic control, in site planning, 14
Orienting building users
    corridor schemes, 19
    helpful facilities, 19
    illus., 19
    use of color, 19
Outpatient department, interior
        planning, 20
Outpatient entrance
    combined with main entrance, 10
    reception control point for, 10
Outpatient drives, design, 10
Outpatient reception desk, direction to, 10
Outpatient traffic patterns
    accessibility, 10
    signs for, 10
Outpatients, separate entrance for, 10

■ ■ ■

Parking
    employee, 12
    multistoried structure. See Parking
        structure
Parking areas
    combined, 12, illus., 12
    location, 12
    related to building entrances, 13
    restrictive signs for, 12
    separated from main entrance drive, 12
    signs for, 12
    in site planning, 15
    traffic movement, 9
Parking structure
    directional signs for, 13
    pedestrian traffic, 15
    reminder signs, 15
Patient care areas, room numbering
        systems, 57-58, illus., 57, 58, 59
Patient floors, interior planning, 21
Patients, served by signs and graphics
        system, 3
Pedestrian access, in site planning, 14

Pedestrian approach route, planning, 7
Pedestrian approaches, location, 11
Pedestrian traffic, parking structure, 15
Pedestrian walkways
    location, 11
    See also Pedestrian approaches
Pictographs
    defined, 37, illus., 37, 38
    examples listed, 39
    standardization, 39-40
    See also Symbols, Terminology
Planning, interior. See Interior planning
Police, served by signs and graphics
        system, 3
Press, served by signs and graphics
        system, 3
Public transportation stops
    approval for posting signs, 11
    signs for, 11
Purchasing signs
    delivery, 54
    specifications, 53
    taking bids and ordering, 53

■ ■ ■

Ramps for the handicapped, 12
Reception control point for outpatient
        entrance, 10
Room numbering, checklist, 34

■ ■ ■

Security checkpoint, near employees'
        entrance, 12
Selection of Architects for Health
        Facility Projects (AHA), 51 n.
Service vehicle area, planning, 7
Service entrance
    secondary drives, 9
    in site planning, 15
Service entrance drive, signs for, 8,
        illus., 8
Sign committee coordinator, responsi-
        bilities, 23
Signs
    acquiring, 51-54
    advisory, 36
    choosing typefaces and design, 41-42
    classification, 36, illus., 36
    costs and budgeting, 52
    delivery and installation, 54
    determining need for, 32
    for hospital identification, 7
    identification, 36, illus., 36
    information, 36
    in-house fabrication, 54
    installation costs, 53
    layout and design, 46-49
    length of message, 48-49
    letter size, 44-45, illus., 45
    limiting number of, 19

    location, 32
    movement, 36
    placement, 50, illus., 50
    precautionary, 36
    purchasing, 53
    related to building site planning, 6
    taking bids and ordering, 53-54
    temporary, 61-62
    typographical legibility, 41-42
    use of color, 40
    written maintenance procedures, 62
Signs and graphics system
    coordinated with new construction
        program, 4
    data collection, 23, 25-26
    development, 23, illus., 24
    development time span, 23, illus., 25
    determining uses and conditions, 25-26
    functions, 3
    maintaining, 61-62
    need for flexibility, 4
    need for hospital building plans, 26
    part of master construction plan, 4
    persons concerned, 23
    publics served, 3-4
    reasons for, 1-2
    sign committee membership, 23
    symbols and pictographs, 37-40,
        illus., 37, 38
    temporary signs, 61-62
    timing, 4
    use of color, 40
Site approach, planning, 7-11
Site planning
    checklist, 14-15
    coordinated with informational
        signs and graphics, 5
Sweet's Architectural Catalog File, 51
Symbols
    distinguished from pictographs, 37
    examples listed, 39
    See also Pictographs, Terminology

■ ■ ■

Temporary signs, need for, 61-62
Terminology, in information system, 35-36
Traffic control, planning, 7-11
Traffic movement, interior planning,
        17-19
Traffic movement patterns, related to
        building design, 5
Traffic patterns
    desirable, 29, illus., 29
    in interior planning, 28-31
    planning modifications, 28-30,
        illus., 30
    trouble spots, 30-31, illus., 30
Trauma center, highway signs, 39
Typefaces
    described, 41-45, illus., 42, 43, 44

legibility in signs, 43-45
weights, 44, illus., 44
Type vocabulary. *See* Typography, basic
terminology
Typography, basic terminology, 41-42

■ ■ ■

User groups
bilingual signs, 25
checklist, 34
determining categories, 25
desirable traffic patterns, 29-30,
illus., 29
handicapped persons, 25-26
in planning for traffic flow, 28-31,
illus., 28
special needs, 34
special requirements, 25

■ ■ ■

Vehicular approach route, planning, 7
Vehicular traffic, movement, 9
Visually handicapped, audible/tactile
signs for, 11
Visitor parking
beyond the drop-off point, 9
planning, 8
signs for, 8
Visitors served by signs and graphics
system, 3
Volunteers served by signs and graphics
system, 4

■ ■ ■

Waiting areas
appropriate facilities, 18-19
near appropriate entrances, 18-19
placement of furnishings, 17, illus., 18
Walkways for pedestrians, 11
Wheelchairs, modified curbs for, 11

■ ■ ■